Beat
Arthritis

Dr. Michael Colgan

For The First Time, The World-Renowned Colgan Institute Reveals Its Program For A Healthy Prostate

www.applepublishing.com

Printed in Canada

FIRST EDITION

Canadian Cataloguing in Publication Data

Colgan, Michael,
       Beat Arthritis

Includes bibliographical references and index.
ISBN: 1-896817-15-7 (bound)
        ISBN: 1-896817-23-8 (pbk.)

       1. Arthritis-Diet therapy. 2. Arthritis-
Nutritional aspects. I. Title

RC933.C643 2000   616.7'220654   C99-900096-9

Apple Publishing Company Ltd.
220 East 59th Avenue
Vancouver, British Columbia
Canada V5X 1X9   Tel: (604) 214-6688   Fax: (604) 214-3566

E-mail: books@applepublishing.com   Web Site: www.applepublishing.com

10   9   8   7   6   5   4   3   2   1

*To my Lesley,
Megan and Tammy
whose constant love
and faith
give me the courage
to seek the truth*

Also by Dr. Michael Colgan:

Electrodermal Responses
The Training Index
Your Personal Vitamin Profile
Prevent Cancer Now
Optimum Sports Nutrition
The New Nutrition: Medicine for the Millennium
Hormonal Health
Protect Your Prostate

www.colganchronicles.com

Forewords

*"Dr. Michael Colgan is synonymous with 'breakthrough research.' This book, **Beat Arthritis**, is another important milestone in his publishing of imperatives in preventative medicine.*

One of my friends, an avid golfer, has had trouble in recent years with arthritis, which he thought was a natural disease of aging. The pain in the joints of his fingers was such that he could not grip his golf clubs to play in his Saturday foursome. After studying Dr. Colgan's work and following his advice, he is almost as good as new. Unfortunately, he is beating me again, just when my confidence was soaring.

Dr. Colgan's laser accurate research and ability to communicate complex scientific data in interesting terms, understandable by the general population, are a brilliant contribution to human health and longevity."

Dr Denis Waitley,
Best-selling author and world recognized speaker,
Author of The Psychology of Winning and Seeds of Greatness

*"This is one of the best health books of the year. It should become a classic and a standard from which to measure health books. Like Dr. Colgan's other books, **Beat Arthritis** reduces the complicated state-of-the-science to understandable concepts that can be put into immediate practice. Dr. Colgan has accurately explained how people can use diet and dietary supplements to make a great difference in their health. He accurately sorts through the maze of research to inform people as to which supplements will best help which arthritic*

v

conditions. As usual, he is ahead of the curve with his practical studies and experience with such new supplements as S-adenosylmethionine (SAMe) for arthritis. Dr. Colgan shows people how they can find natural and safe relief from both osteoarthritis and rheumatoid arthritis."

Dr Richard Passwater,
Renowned researcher and author of more than 50 books on nutrition

"I have eagerly anticipated Dr. Colgan's publication of **Beat Arthritis.** I'm not disappointed. This is an incisive, easily understood and invaluable source of information for arthritis sufferers and health professionals from the leading expert in the new science of wellness."

Dr Charles Myers,
Physician, British Columbia, Canada

"Dr. Colgan's research is outstanding. Coupled with this, his wonderfully understandable explanations and practical applications make his books excellent tools for physicians and patients alike. Congratulations Michael on another essential literary work for our time and beyond."

Dr Jackie Mills,
Physician, Auckland, New Zealand

Acknowledgments

The great people I work with urged me to take time out from my schedule in order to write this book. The great scientists and physicians whose work is documented herein gave me the knowledge. Together they aided me beyond measure to find my way through the complicated maze of physiology, biochemistry and nutrition, to commit to print what the Colgan Institute has been doing since 1974 to help people protect their joints.

Whenever I lapsed into the obscure language of science, my staff on the project brought me back to reality with a sharp KISS. "Keep it simple stupid." In tribute to their help in writing a plain and simple story, I salute the unfailing wit and wisdom of Marion Halliwell (who processed every word), Cheryl Harrison, Eric Booth, Jocelyn Pettigrew, Aileen Speight, Steven Macramallah and my wife and lifelong scientific colleague of the eagle eye, Lesley Colgan.

Thanks also to my colleagues who generously suspended other work we are doing together to give me the space to complete the book, and to all those who have allowed me to use their aching joints as guinea pigs to test my nutritional notions.

And loving thanks to my daughters Megan and Tammy, who crept down the corridor and muffled their dogs whenever "Dads" was ensconced in his study, chuntering and grumbling in the throes of giving birth.

Introduction

Joint and connective tissue disorders, from osteoarthritis, rheumatoid arthritis and gout to fibromyalgia and chronic fatigue syndrome, are now the most prevalent forms of disability in Western Society. Joint and soft tissue injuries are also the most common problems that prevent athletes from reaching their potential, and are major causes of a premature end to many athletic careers. For more than two decades, the Colgan Institute has been developing a system for tackling these problems.

As we enter the new millennium, I am making this system available to everyone because of a fundamental shift that is occurring in the medical treatment of arthritis and other joint disorders. For more than a century, the major medical approach has been a mask of symptomatic relief, an obsolete medicine that allows the illness to progress beneath the mask and even accelerates that progression. Only in the last five years have physicians generally recognized that the way to long-lasting help for their patients is to provide the body with the structural materials required to re-build damaged joints. We have been trying to do that at the Colgan Institute since 1974. I hope that many physicians and many thousands of their patients may benefit from our experience.

Michael Colgan, PhD
Saltspring Island
British Columbia
August 1999

Contents

New Facts, New Focus

Many folk think of arthritis as only three diseases, **osteoarthritis, rheumatoid arthritis,** and **gout.** In fact it's a term used to describe hundreds of different degenerative disorders, from multiple forms of lupus, ankylosing spondylitis, Chrohn's disease, and bursitis to arthritis caused by trauma and by infectious agents such as tuberculosis, Lyme disease, and Epstein-Barr virus, to the modern disorders of fibromyalgia and chronic fatigue. They all involve progressive stiffness, swelling, tenderness, pain, deformity, and loss of motion in the joints. In June 1999, the Centers for Disease Control reported that arthritis is the leading cause of disability in the United States, affecting 43 million people. [1]

The Man Upstairs had little regard for gender equality when handing out arthritis. The numerous types of rheumatoid arthritis attack three times as many women as men. After age 45, the even more numerous types of osteoarthritis attack *ten* times as many women as men. As our analysis progresses you will see why women are so afflicted and what they can do to prevent it.

Only with gout do men outnumber women. About 95% of cases of the various forms of gout are male. But pure cases of gout are rare, affecting fewer than three men in every 1000.[2,3] Nevertheless, this book has to cover gout because it is often a contributing disease in other forms of arthritis, and often overlooked in diagnosis and treatment. Many cases of arthritis of the hands, for example, one of the most common disorders of aging, are now known to be at least two diseases, gout and osteoarthritis.[3,4] Treating only one or the other is doomed to failure.

We will see that most cases of arthritis are similarly mixed bags. The overlapping and intermittent symptoms of the various diseases involved, make the individual patient's problem incredibly difficult to analyze by the usual medical tests, thus almost impossible to treat successfully with conventional, drug-oriented medicine.

In the diseases respectively called osteoarthritis and rheumatoid arthritis, for example, the dominant clinical findings may be joint deformity, loss of motion, and degeneration of cartilage (the pads of soft tissue that cushion your joints).[2,3] Inflammation and elevated levels of components of the immune system, such as tumor necrosis factor (TNF) — two symptoms that are used to distinguish rheumatoid from osteo conditions — may be variously present or absent depending on the time of test.

Obsolete Treatment

Consequently, the usual medical answer to arthritis today is still symptomatic relief — aspirin or other **non-steroidal anti-inflammatory drugs (NSAIDs)** — little different from the treatment of 100 years ago. These drugs make the patient temporarily more comfortable, but do nothing to stop the progress of the disease. In fact, as clinical studies have shown for 20 years, and as most physicians now know, long-term use of aspirin and other NSAIDs prevents your body from repairing cartilage, and thus *accelerates* the progression of arthritis.[6,7]

As arthritis progresses, medicine has little else to offer, except even more destructive drugs, such as **corticosteroids, gold salts, hydroxychloroquine,** and the cancer chemotherapy drug **methotrexate**. The inevitable final failure of these foibles results in death of the affected joints and their eventual replacement with crude, robotic chunks of alien metal. As owners of these foreign joints will tell you privately, they are at best a hobbledehoy solution.

But times they are a-changin'. As we enter the new millennium, the medical focus on arthritis is shifting to *prevention and cure.* Intensive research in the last decade of this century shows that maintenance and restoration of the cellular matrix of membrane, cartilage and bone, should replace drugs as the principle intervention.

By examining the processes of cellular biology that produce optimum health, I will show you why the use of drugs provides a measure of symptomatic relief, yet worsens the disease. I will show you also how drugs worsen existing widespread nutritional deficiencies, and create new deficiencies that accelerate the main degenerative processes in arthritis — the progressive destruction of the ends of the bones and of the membranes and cartilage between joints.[2,3] And I will show you how to overcome these problems for life.

As I have documented elsewhere, cellular integrity is largely dependent on a continuing supply of the correct structural materials to build new cells.[8] These materials come only from the nutrients you eat, and the biochemicals that your body, unhindered by drugs, can make from these nutrients. If you have arthritis, or even if you are just getting a little creaky, you need to read this book from cover to cover before you put another morsel into your mouth.

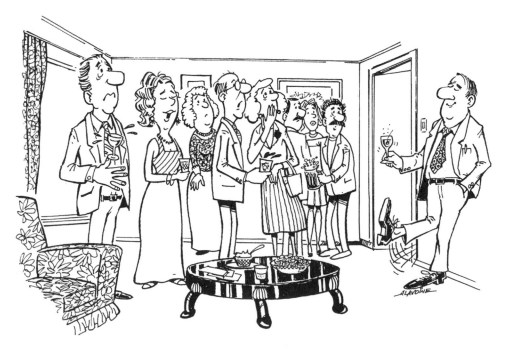

"Henry loves grossing people out since they put his knee joint in backwards!"

Lean and Clean

If I am correct that eating the right structural materials to maintain your joints can beat arthritis, we should see wide variations in the incidence of arthritis in societies with different diets. And we do. The disorders classified as rheumatoid arthritis, for example, are almost non-existent in traditional societies that eat our ancestral diet of organic whole grains, fresh vegetables, fruits and essential fats, with little meat, low saturated fats, low sugar, low refined carbohydrates and few man-made chemicals.[1,2]

The specific dietary variables that prevent rheumatoid arthritis are difficult to tease out of such a complex nutritional mix, but one critical factor is clear. Studies show unequivocally that traditional diets are high in essential omega-3 and omega-6 fats and modern diets are very low in essential fats. These nutrients are so important in beating arthritis, I give each a chapter ahead.

Out, Out Saturated Fat

A second important difference between traditional and modern diets is the high level of saturated fat we eat in meats and dairy foods.   We don't know whether this fat causes rheumatoid arthritis directly, but studies show that saturated fat in the diet definitely worsens rheumatoid disorders.[3]   As documented in some of my other books, saturated fat disrupts the metabolism of essential fats. This disruption is one likely mechanism by which it promotes arthritis.[4,5]

So, get the saturated fat out of your diet.   Also, avoid all processed vegetable oils and margarines, and all foods containing hydrogenated or partially hydrogenated fats.   Processing and hydrogenation create *trans* fats, toxic compounds that are equivalent to saturated fats in the damage they do to your body.[4]

Avoid Red Meats: Eat Fish

Meats, especially red meats, are not only high in saturated fats, but also contain high levels of arachidonic acid. This preformed omega-6 fat is the precursor of a highly inflammatory compound in your body called **Prostaglandin E$_2$**. Folk who eat high levels of red meats are likely to create a pro-inflammatory condition in all their tissues.

At the Colgan Institute, we did a one-year series of case studies on strength athletes who ate large amounts of red meat as their main source of protein, and who also suffered frequent joint problems.   Every one of them had abnormally high levels of arachidonic acid in their blood.   When we took them off red meat and substituted ion-exchange whey protein concentrate as their main protein source, arachidonic acid levels declined and joint problems diminished. Controlled studies report similar results in patients with rheumatoid arthritis.[6]

Another good protein source is fish (except certain species, listed in Table 1 on page 11). Research is uncovering strong links between a high fish protein diet and protection against arthritis. In the latest study, Dr J A Shapiro and team at the University of Washington in Seattle showed that even two meals of baked or broiled fish per week dramatically reduced the risk of rheumatoid arthritis in women.[7]

So fish is in and red meat is definitely out if you want to beat arthritis. An occasional chop will not hurt if you just can't resist. But waving your butcher good day from the other side of the street is sound medicine for your joints. Whenever the thought of a juicy steak sets the saliva a-flowing, remember, be kind to your knees, you'll miss them when they're gone.

Get Your Veggies

Traditional societies that show a low incidence of many "Western" diseases, typically have high intakes of both cooked and uncooked, organically-grown vegetables. Even in Western and Westernized countries, numerous studies show that high vegetable intake lowers the risk of atherosclerosis, numerous forms of cancer, and some other diseases.[8] Until now, however, high vegetable intake has not been studied extensively in relation to arthritis. As we might suspect, the link is unmistakable.

The newest research, published in March 1998, is representative of recent findings. Dr C La Vecchia and colleagues at the Institute for Pharmacological Research in Milan, Italy, examined the frequency of vegetable consumption in a representative sample of 50,000 Italians. They found that high intakes of vegetables reduced the risk of a wide variety of diseases, especially arthritis.[9]

Research aimed directly at arthritis confirms the power of vegetables. In a representative study at the National Hospital Institute of Rheumatology in Oslo, Norway, rheumatoid arthritis patients were put on a vegetarian diet for one year and compared with a control group. Fourteen of the fifteen measures showed better control of symptoms with the vegetable-based diet.[10]

In an even more specific trial, Dr M T Nenonen and colleagues at the University of Kuopio in Finland, studied the effect of an uncooked vegetable diet on rheumatoid arthritis. Such a diet is high in **unprocessed chlorophyllins, antioxidant flavonoids, fiber,** and **live lactobacilli,** some of the beneficial microorganisms that populate the human gut. Results showed a significant decrease in disease activity, so much so that patients were able to stop their gold, methotrexate, and other drugs. When patients returned to their usual diets, their arthritis returned also.[11]

Research to date has pinpointed only a few of the substances in vegetables that help to beat arthritis.[4,8,12]   In Chapter 11 Antioxidants Against Arthritis, I cover some of them and in discussions of essential fats, vitamins and fermented yoghurt, I cover others. But the evidence is clear that a high intake of mixed vegetables, both raw and lightly cooked, provides other nutrients, and nutrient interactions yet unknown to science, that help to protect your joints.

Gout Is Everywhere

Gout occurs when crystals of **uric acid** invade the joints. The major cause of gout is **hyperuricaemia,** high levels of uric acid in the blood. Uric acid is a normal component of your body but becomes toxic when serum levels rise above about six milligrams per 100 milliliters. By seven milligrams per 100 milliliters, sharp crystals are forming in your joints. They cause excruciating pain, especially to joints rich in nerves, such as the big toe.

Remember the Victorian caricature of gout and over-indulgence — a wealthy man with an alcoholic face, his heavily bandaged foot set up on a cushion. Though the comic portrayal has disappeared, the disease of gout continues to plague Western Society. It is even on the increase.[13] Overall, about 20% of the US population has hyperuricaemia, and are at risk of uric acid crystals invading their joints.[14]

We know now that these crystals commonly occur simultaneously with other forms of arthritis. Increasing numbers of studies urge rheumatologists to test for joint infiltration, as an additional disease entity involved in both rheumatoid and osteo forms of arthritis.[15,16] I suspect that the same gouty complications will also be found when researchers look for them in arthritic forms of fibromyalgia and chronic fatigue syndrome.

Self-Induced Agony

Like the over-indulgent Victorian gentleman, prostrate in agony, most folk who get urate crystals in their joints do it all to themselves. The majority of cases of hyperuricaemia occur from two causes: ingestion of edibles that increase bodily production of uric acid, and ingestion of edibles that reduce the body's ability to excrete uric acid in urine via the kidneys.[17]

Foods high in **purines** will raise uric acid levels in almost anyone. The worst offender is beer. Not only is its purine content over the moon, but the alcohol and other chemicals in beer also inhibit uric acid excretion from the body.[18,19] Some arthritics believe they can dodge this problem by drinking low-alcohol or alcohol-free beers. Can't be done. Recent research shows that all forms of beer raise uric acid levels and inhibit its excretion.[19]

Distilled liquors are almost as bad because of their high alcohol content. So is red wine because of a multitude of chemicals it contains. White wine in moderation is the best, but still does nothing to reduce uric acid levels.

In contrast, plain water dramatically increases purine and urate excretion from the body.[19] Not only for gouty problems, but for many reasons, a steady intake of 10 - 12 glasses of pure water every day is a key component of our beat arthritis program.

More high purine foods are given in Table 1, together with other foods that raise uric acid levels. Especially important to avoid are refined carbohydrates, including all white flour products, white and enriched flour breads and baked goods. Although not high in purines, these foods will send your uric acid into the stratosphere. So will the sugar **fructose**.[20] Saturated fats and *trans* fats also raise uric acid levels because they inhibit its excretion.[21]

Table 1. Foods high in purines and other edibles that raise uric acid levels

Beer	Herring
Red meats	Sardines
All organ meats (heart, liver,	Anchovies
kidneys, sweetbreads, brains)	Fish roe
Patés	Caviar
All types of beans	Mussels
Liquor	Aged cheeses
Red wine	Fructose
Cocktails	Saturated fats
Port	Refined carbohydrates
Liqueurs	Diuretic drugs

© 1998, The Colgan Institute, San Diego, CA

A final common cause of deposition of crystals in the joints is prescription drugs. The worst offenders are diuretics which inhibit excretion of uric acid via the kidneys.[15] If you have arthritis and your uric acid level is above 5.5 milligrams per 100 milliliters, and you are using prescribed diuretics for another problem such as water retention or hypertension, take this book and the medical references to your physician. Alternative medication could save you a lot of suffering.

To end on a happy note, one nutrient that dramatically lowers uric acid by inhibiting the bodily enzyme necessary for making it, is the essential vitamin **folic acid**. Chapters ahead cover other benefits for arthritis from this remarkable nutrient, but prevention of gout alone warrants its use every day. A dose of two milligrams of folic acid combined with 200 micrograms of vitamin B_{12} is a Godsend![22]

The Anti-Arthritis Diet

To summarize this chapter in one sentence, to avoid arthritis eat our ancestral diet. Specifically:

- **Eat whole grains**, not refined carbohydrates.

- **Eat fresh vegetables**, not canned or preserved. Avoid all beans.

- **Eat fresh fruits**, not canned, dried or preserved.

- **Eat fish first, then white meat**, not red meats. Avoid organ meats, certain fish and fish roe.

- **Eat a low-fat diet**, especially avoid aged cheeses.

- **Eat essential fats**, not saturated or *trans* fats.

- **Eat a low-sugar diet**, especially avoid fructose.

- If you must, **drink white wine**, not beer, liquor or red wine.

- **Drink 10 – 12 glasses of water** every day.

- **Avoid man-made chemicals**, especially diuretic drugs.

- **Eat moderately**. Keep that bodyfat at bay.

- Make your diet and your body **lean and clean**.

Some folk referred to the Colgan Institute have called this regimen strict. So it may seem at the beginning. But as arthritis fades away and you feel the multiple benefits, it is no more onerous than cleaning your teeth, and a much bigger benefit to your health. After about a year, when symptoms disappear, you can be confident you have transformed your body. Thereafter, moderate indulgence in forbidden foods will no longer send you running for the aspirin.

> *A healthy body is a guest-chamber for the soul, a sick body a prison.*
> *Victor Hugo*

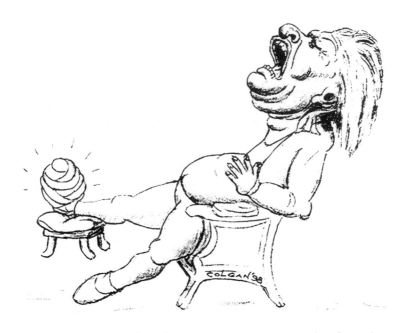

The weariest and most burdened route
Is paradise beside the gout.

Omega-3 Fats Whack Arthritis

Western diets are woefully deficient in essential fats, especially omega-3 fats. As documented in my book **Essential Fats,** 80% of folk in America, Canada, Australia and New Zealand are short of omega-3s.[1] Correction of just this one dietary deficiency has dramatic benefits for rheumatoid arthritis disorders.

The benefits of the **omega-3 fats** in flax oil for treatment of arthritis were first outlined by Dr Johanna Budwig in 1959 in Zurich, Switzerland.[2] Budwig's brilliant analysis, however, was largely ignored in America because all her papers were in German, and unlike their European colleagues, American scientists usually know only one language.

It was not until the '80s that Dr Joel Kremer of Albany Medical College in New York, gave fish oil omega-3s to rheumatoid arthritis patients. Without any other nutritional changes, the omega-3 fats alone reduced inflammation, pain, and tenderness of arthritic joints by 50%.[3] Since then, more than 20 double-blind, placebo-controlled studies have confirmed Kremer's findings.[4-7]

The omega-3 in fish oil most responsible for these benefits is **eicosapentaenoic acid**. Whether or not you eat oily fish such as salmon, your body makes eicosapentaenoic acid out of the essential vegetable fat alpha-linolenic acid. The sequence of conversion of essential fats is shown in Figure 1.[1]

It Takes A Lot Of Fish Oil

You have to take a lot of omega-3s to get the optimum effect. Successful studies have used 60 – 130 milligrams per kilogram bodyweight per day.[6] At the upper end, that's 10 grams a day for a 175 pound (80 kg) man and eight grams a day for a 120 pound (55 kg) woman. The best fish oil is only 50% omega-3 fats, so it takes double the amount of oil to provide the dose. That's 20 of the largest capsules (1000 mg) per day for the man and 16 capsules for the woman, enough to choke a horse.

At the Colgan Institute, for those who prefer fish oil we use a dose of 60 milligrams per kilogram per day. That's 10 capsules for the male example and eight capsules for the female.

For most folk, however, compliance is still difficult because of the large number of horse pills to swallow, or the foul taste of fish oil if taken as a liquid. Fish oil is also expensive, and if bought in bulk to save money, poses the risk of the highly biologically active oil going rancid, even in capsule form.[8] Lucky for us there is a more palatable alternative.

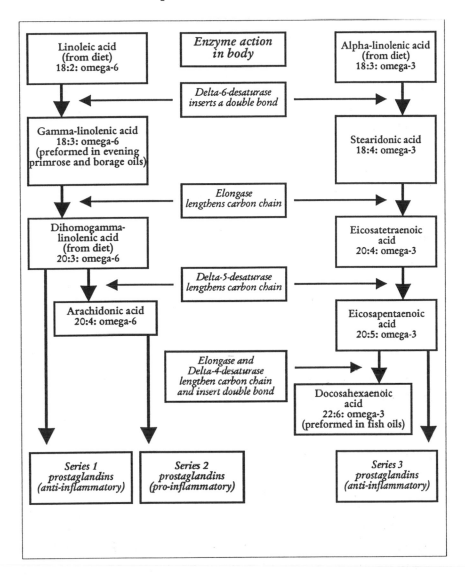

Figure 1. How the human body converts essential fats to fats with special functions.

Flax Oil Works

Recent studies, which returned to the use of flax oil as specified by Budwig, show that it raises blood levels of **eicosapentaenoic acid** in arthritis patients just as well as fish oil.[9] Eicosapentaenoic acid is the most important omega-3 fat in fish oils. Flax oil does not contain eicosapentaenoic acid, but your body converts the omega-3 fats in flax oil into eicosapentaenoic acid very nicely. Flax oil, at equivalent doses to fish oil, also reduces inflammation, tenderness and morning stiffness.[9,10] It's less costly and less subject to spoilage.

One problem with flax oil is the dose needed for the body to convert to eicosapentaenoic acid sufficient for folk with confirmed arthritis. Most books and articles I have read recommend far too little. Flax oil is 45 - 55% omega-3 fats depending on the flax variety, soil, weather and other factors that influence the composition of oils in growing plants. We take 50% as an average. Our analysis of all relevant research indicates that only about a quarter of the omega-3s in flax oil survive the journey through digestion, absorption, and conversion to eicosapentaenoic acid by your body. Consequently, to provide an effective five grams increase in blood eicosapentaenoic acid for a 175 pound (80 kg) person, requires 40 grams of flax oil (two large tablespoons).

For such a large daily dose, it's a boon that properly extracted organic flax oil is available today from Barlean's, Omega, Flora and Arrowhead Mills. These brands are very palatable in salad dressings, milk shakes and other foods, recipes for which are given in Appendix A, Gourmet Foods for Joints.

One special food deserves mention. Dr Johanna Budwig was the first to recognize that flax oil mixed with lightly fermented low-fat cottage cheese, a food called **quark,** improves the absorption and utilization of essential fats.[2] Flavored with fruit or savory tastes, it makes a great lunch dish. If you use flax oil with quark, we calculate you can reduce the dose by 25%, to 1½ tablespoons a day.

The Odd Minority

About 10% of arthritis patients don't seem to be able to make sufficient eicosapentaenoic acid, no matter how much flax oil they take. Various factors, such as saturated fats or *trans* fats in their diets, inhibit an enzyme in the body called **delta-6-desaturase**, which is essential for conversion of the alpha-linolenic acid in flax oil into eicosapentaenoic acid.

Folk affected in this way are often hard to identify without extensive testing. So, to increase the efficacy of omega-3 treatment of arthritis, in all cases we use some fish oil together with the flax oil. Vegetarians can use eicosapentaenoic acid from the sea vegetable **nori.**

How much fish oil or nori oil to take depends on the individual's willingness to swallow large capsules. We find that six capsules a day is usually the limit. These supply about three grams of eicosapentaenoic acid, leaving the balance of the dose to be provided by flax oil. Confused? Don't be. The exact program is given in Chapter 13.

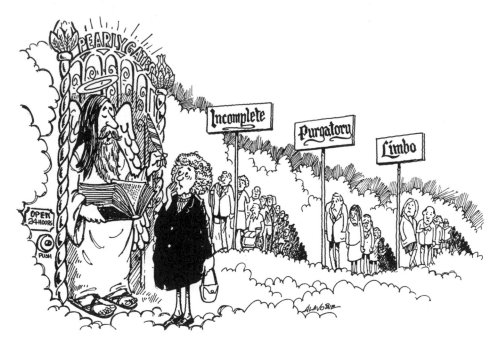

"No I'm sorry, false hips won't do. It says here we sent you down with all your parts.
You'll have to wait in the incomplete line until we find your hip joints!"

4

Omega-6 Fats Whack Arthritis

Gamma-linolenic acid (GLA), the omega-6 fat found most plentifully in **borage oil,** also benefits arthritis, especially the various forms of rheumatoid arthritis. In animal studies, and at least 10 controlled clinical trials with human subjects, GLA reduces arthritic symptoms of morning stiffness, joint pain, swelling and tenderness by 25 – 50%.[1,2]

One of the latest studies illustrates an important principle of all nutritional healing. Arthritis patients treated with GLA for six months showed a 25% improvement in symptoms. Not spectacular, but the smart researchers then carried on the study a further six months. Improvements were progressive over the whole period.[3] Whenever you adopt a nutritional strategy, you have to give the body time to grow sufficient new, improved tissues in the enriched nutritional environment, to enable healing to occur.

Borage and Pumpkin Oils Best

Largely because of the persuasive writings of Dr David Horrobin, most studies of GLA and arthritis have used **evening primrose oil**. Unfortunately, this strategy limits the practical dosage because, despite its popularity as a supplement, evening primrose oil is only 9% GLA. So to obtain the effective dose of about 2.5 grams GLA for a 175 pound (80 kg) person, patients have to take 28 of the 1000 milligram horse pills. Faced with this mountain of capsules every day, compliance disappears faster 'n a bug in a blender.

Other studies have used **blackcurrant seed oil**,[4] which is about 17% GLA (omega-6) and about 15% omega-3. Trying to get both omega-6 and omega-3 fats into the same capsule, they fail to get an adequate dose of either. To obtain sufficient eicosapentaenoic acid, which we saw in Chapter 3 can take five grams of omega-3 fats, would require a whopping 34 capsules of blackcurrant oil per day. To obtain sufficient GLA (omega-six fats) from this source requires a still unacceptable 15 capsules per day.

At 24%, **borage oil** contains the highest concentration of GLA and is my choice as the best source. But you still need a good source of linoleic acid, which, in most folk, will readily convert to GLA.

Well informed readers may object that evening primrose, blackcurrant and borage oils also contain 71%, 48%, and 40% respectively of linoleic acid, and that a large proportion of this would convert to GLA. So it would if the individual's delta-6-desaturase enzyme is working well to do the conversion. But these exotic oils are extremely expensive sources of linoleic acid, up to 100 times the cost of walnut or pumpkin seed oils which are respectively 50% and 45% linoleic acid. Even at only 14% linoleic acid, flax oil is a much less expensive source.

At the Colgan Institute, we use **organic pumpkin seed oil**, which is 45% linoleic acid, as the main source of linoleic acid to convert in the body to GLA. But, as with the omega-3 fats, to allow for those folk whose conversion enzymes are compromised, we add whatever number of borage oil capsules the person will tolerate and adjust the dosage accordingly.

All this dosage gobbledegook will become crystal clear ahead, when you reach the overall strategy to beat arthritis in Chapter 13. But to comprehend how each step of that strategy works, first you should know the mechanisms by which omega-6 and omega-3 fats combat arthritis.

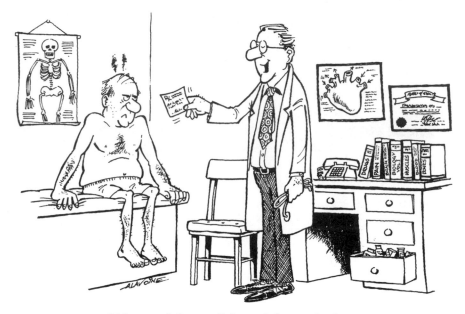

*"This prescription won't do much for your back,
but it's cheap and has a great array of side effects!"*

Essential Fats Combat Inflammation

The first way in which GLA (omega-6) and eicosapentaenoic acid (omega-3) combat arthritis, is by increasing bodily production of the anti-inflammatory compounds called **prostaglandin E_1** and **prostaglandin E_3**, and reducing production of the pro-inflammatory **prostaglandin E_2**. Researchers at the University of Strathclyde in Glasgow, Scotland, have recently shown these effects, both in arthritis patients and in healthy volunteers.[1]

But the actions of these golden oils extend far beyond this simple paradigm. The omega-3 fats from flax oil and fish oil also inhibit other inflammatory actions of the human immune system, and reduce auto-immune damage.[1,2] They also directly modify pain, so much so that many patients can eliminate their use of aspirin use of aspirin and other NSAIDs.[2,3] This effect stops the progressive destruction of cartilage by NSAIDs, and opens a very important treatment window for nutritional strategies that assist cartilage to regenerate.

The GLA from borage oil and from conversion of pumpkin seed oil also has further beneficial actions. One of the big problems in rheumatoid conditions is the body attacking itself, via the immune system, with **tumor necrosis factor** (TNF). This immune system soldier, named for its ability to kill cancer cells, also destroys cartilage, membrane and bone. GLA directly inhibits the TNF attack.[1]

Unlike omega-3 fats, GLA also suppresses **synovitis** in rheumatoid conditions.[4] Synovitis is inflammation of the synovial membrane of the joint socket. This inflammation not only causes pain directly but also reduces the production of synovial fluid by the membrane. Synovial fluid is critical to healthy joints, as it is the lubrication between surfaces that allows them to slide as the joint moves. The increase in lubrication alone is ample justification for using omega-6 fats.

Rebuilding Your Joints

Although essential fats provide significant relief from symptoms of arthritis, and also provide some of the nutrient components of joint and cartilage structure, their use alone is only a little better than the usual medical treatment of symptoms. Why? Because they do not rebuild degenerated cartilage or synovial membranes, or the degenerated ends of bones. Essential fats relieve the pain, reduce inflammation and eliminate the use of NSAIDs. By doing so they set the stage for joint repair, so that the main nutritional components can perform their miraculous dance.

The cartilage between your joints contains cells called **chondrocytes** which continuously renew worn out bits. Chondrocytes achieve this magic by producing strong, feathery threads called **proteoglycans,** and strings of collagen called **collagen fibrils.** These components knit together to form a tough but spongy cushion of cartilage that reduces the shock of bone bumping on bone, and stops the ends of the bones rubbing each other raw.

The cartilage cushion is lubricated by **synovial fluid,** "joint oil", which enables the joints to slide effortlessly through their range of motion. Synovial fluid is produced by the **synovial membrane**, a slippery sheath which lines the **joint capsule**. The capsule itself is a strong, inelastic sleeve that seals the whole joint to the ends of the bones. Figure 2 illustrates the basic structure.

Any of three main conditions initiate and perpetuate arthritis:

- The rate of destruction of the cartilage exceeds the body's capacity to replace it.

- Inflammation of the synovial membrane inhibits production of synovial fluid (joint oil).

- Toxic substances, such as uric acid, get into the joint.

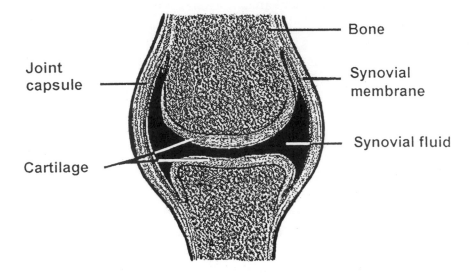

Figure 2. Basic structure of a joint

Once essential fats have set the stage by inhibiting inflammation, pain, and attacks by the immune system, and eliminating the need for NSAIDs, the main goals of therapy are to provide the structural components that enable the joint to produce sufficient cartilage and synovial fluid to repair and maintain itself. That's our next step to beat arthritis.

> *As Pooh might say,*
> *"Take 'specially good care of your hips.*
> *It's awfully uncomfortable to have to bump*
> *downstairs on your bottom."*

6

Glucosamine Forms Half The Structure

Glucosamine is an essential structural component of proteoglycans, the strong feathery threads made by the chondrocytes, that knit your cartilage together. Glucosamine is the rate-limiting chemical step in proteoglycans production. Hence, together with the collagen fibrils also produced by the chondrocytes, glucosamine determines the rate at which you can replace cartilage. The basic structure of cartilage is shown in Figure 3.

Your body makes glucosamine from glucose and the amino acid **glutamine,** using an enzyme called **glucosamine synthetase.** For unknown reasons, activity of this enzyme declines with aging, thereby limiting glucosamine production. When the rate of glucosamine production falls below that required to maintain the supply of proteoglycans, arthritis begins.

Even if the glucosamine synthetase enzyme is operating normally, glucosamine production may be compromised by an insufficient supply of glutamine, because glutamine is in constant demand by your muscles, immune system and joints. My book, **Optimum Sports Nutrition,** documents how athletic training alone can easily overwhelm your glutamine supply.[1]

Structure of Cartilage

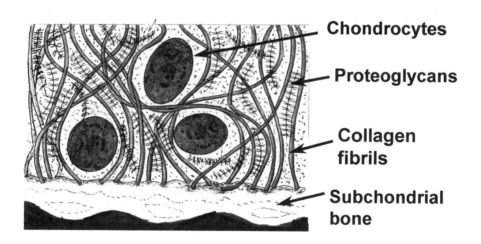

Figure 3. The basic structure of cartilage

Maintain Your Muscle

Glutamine is made mainly in your muscles. The amount you can make depends on how much muscle you have. The usual loss of muscle with age, especially in women, seriously compromises their glutamine supply. That's a major reason why all our programs at the Colgan Institute include weight bearing exercise. The right exercise plus sufficient protein can easily maintain muscle lifelong. An effective exercise program is outlined in Chapter 14.

Glutamine is made from the essential branched-chain amino acids, **isoleucine, leucine** and **valine,** which you have to obtain from protein foods. Insufficient protein or poor quality protein in the diet also compromises body glutamine. So folk with arthritis should be especially careful to get the right protein. As I have documented elsewhere, ion-exchange and cross-flow membrane extraction whey proteins have the highest Biological Value, the best measure of the amount of protein retained in the body.[1] Sources and brands are given in Chapter 13.

Finally, your immune system cannot make glutamine, yet cannot make a move without it. So, in order to maintain immunity, your body makes heavy demands every day on your muscle to supply glutamine. These demands can easily leave insufficient glutamine for the joints. Without enough glutamine to make the glucosamine necessary for proteoglycans, arthritis is inevitable.

Fortunately you can offset this glucosamine shortage with glucosamine supplements. These provide extra glucosamine to the joints, ready-made for the production of proteoglycans. Animal studies show that oral **glucosamine sulfate** can increase proteoglycans production by up to 170%.[2,3]

Clinical Benefits of Glucosamine

A pile of controlled studies since 1980 show that the increase in proteoglycans, caused by glucosamine supplements, has big clinical benefits. I can cover only a smidgen of the research in this little book, so I will cite examples that show you the trend of evidence.

A representative study of subjects with arthritic knees was done by Dr Anthonio Vaz Lopez at St Johns Hospital in Oporto, Portugal. In a double-blind trial, he gave patients either 1.5 grams of glucosamine or 1.2 grams of **ibuprofen**. By the end of the research, the glucosamine subjects had significantly less pain and greater return of function than the ibuprofen group.[14]

In another study comparing glucosamine to an inert placebo, a group of arthritic patients was given only 500 milligrams of glucosamine daily for just 14 days. The placebo group showed no change in condition, whereas the glucosamine group showed a 70% reduction in pain and swelling, plus a large increase in joint function.[14]

Glucosamine also works to overcome cartilage damage in athletes. In a representative study, 51 male and 17 female athletes with cartilage injuries in the knees, were given 1500 milligrams of glucosamine sulfate daily for 40 days, then 750 milligrams daily for another 100 days. Of the 68 athletes, 52 showed *complete cure* of their injury and resumed full training. A follow-up 12 months later showed no signs of cartilage damage in any of them.[15]

All of the convincing studies with glucosamine have used **glucosamine sulfate**. You will see products for sale using other forms such as glucosamine HCl, but despite all sorts of fancy claims, they don't work nearly as well. The sulfate form was adopted in the first place precisely because sulfur is an essential component of glucosamine in the manufacture of proteoglycans.[3]

Over the last decade at the Colgan Institute, we have used up to five grams of glucosamine sulfate per day with hundreds of athletes and arthritis patients. In controlled case studies using glucosamine in conjunction with essential fats, plus sports massage and rehabilitative exercises, we see a success rate, judged by return to full activity, of over 60%. This is a better rate by far than can be achieved by any combination of over-the-counter medications or prescription drugs.

But before you even think of trying these supplements, read the medical references given. You can obtain abstracts easily from the Internet by dialing into the medical libraries at Internet Grateful Med (http://igm.nlm.nih.gov). Then take this book and the references to your physician. If he or she doesn't appear to be listening, be patient. Until they digest the hard evidence, some physicians suffer badly from pharmaceutical fluff in the ears.

There was an old man from Killeet,
Who ate two great buckets of meat,
Washed down with sweet wine,
The best of the vine,
Now he can't lift his nose
from his feet.

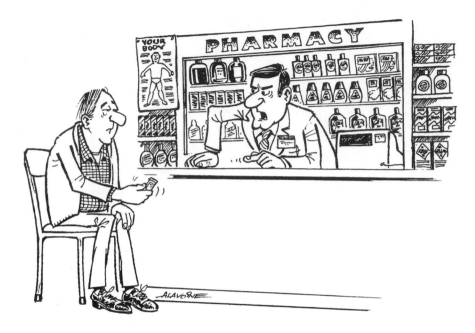

"Of course it says " KEEP TIGHTLY CLOSED," but you are
allowed to open it to get the pills out!"

The Chondroitin Dilemma

Chondroitin is another important biochemical manufactured in your joints. In conjunction with sulfur, it forms a big part of the proteoglycans structure of cartilage. It acts also to assist synovial fluid to lubricate the cartilage.

Chondroitin and synovial fluid both decline in numerous arthritic disorders. The cartilage loses bulk and progressively dries out, becoming stiff and scratchy like a kitchen scouring pad.[1] The sliding surfaces eventually become like sandpaper, especially if crystals of uric acid, calcium pyrophosphate or other minerals have infiltrated the joint. So it is a reasonable idea to try to overcome these problems with supplements of **chondroitin sulfate**.

Trouble is, chondroitin sulfate has a hard job getting through your intestinal wall and into the bloodstream. With a molecular weight of about 30,000 for most preparations of the compound, the chondroitin molecule is far too big. In contrast, glucosamine sulfate has a molecular weight of just 211, and passes through the wall like ants up a trouser leg.

Animal studies in the 1980's, using radioactively-labeled chondroitin, showed increased levels of radioactivity in the blood, suggesting that it was somehow getting through.[2,3] This work led to wild claims for chondroitin as the answer to arthritis, and it's distribution worldwide as a nutritional supplement. More sophisticated recent work on rabbits and on human subjects, however, shows negligible absorption of *intact* chondroitin.[1,4,5]

Nevertheless, studies with rats and men, using oral doses of radioactively-labeled chondroitin, continue to show increases in the blood of chondroitin-related and proteoglycan-related molecules.[6] Many of these molecules are still too big to have passed in from the gut. Most likely they are reconstructed in the blood from small molecular components which are released from chondroitin when it is broken down by digestion. One of these small components is glucosamine sulfate. Your body performs this construction miracle continually with many of the nutrients you eat every day.

Research with new, more sensitive methods of analysis support the idea that the body does reconstruct components of chondroitin. In a representative study, Dr L Silvestro and colleagues at Res Pharma in Torino, Italy, examined the changes in blood proteoglycans in healthy men, after oral doses of chondroitin sulfate. They showed that numerous proteoglycan-like substances appeared in the blood. They also showed that some of these substances had lost their sulfur content, indicating that they had been broken down and separated from the sulfur, most likely in the gut, and then reconstructed without sulfur in the blood. [7] It is feasible that these pre-formed chunks of proteoglycans could flow to the joints and be used to increase the proteoglycans of cartilage.

More Chondroitin Benefits

Other recent studies show two more beneficial effects of oral chondroitin sulfate. It can raise blood levels of another important compound called **hyaluronan**, a sticky gel that cements the tissues together in your joints. [8]   Chondroitin can also increase normal collagen formation in joints, a very difficult task. Remember, we saw earlier that collagen fibrils and proteoglycans together form the structure of cartilage. [9,10]

Some popular articles suggest that collagen in joints can be increased easily by taking chicken gelatin or collagen extracted from cows. I wish it were so. The latest research shows no beneficial effects of these folk remedies on arthritis. [11]

I have been skeptical of chondroitin in earlier writings, and have thought that its reliable, though moderate effects[12] were a result of the glucosamine it released. With the considerable new evidence, I have to bow, always, to science and amend my view. Although it may not be absorbed intact, there are benefits of chondroitin for arthritis in addition to those conferred by glucosamine. [9,10]

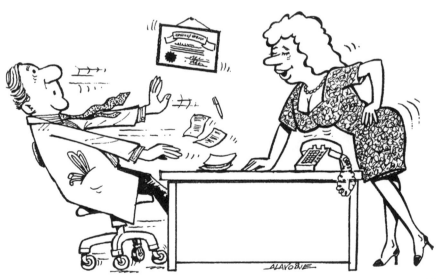

Patient: "The SAMe gives me so much energy Dr. Darling, but I'm single!"
Doctor: "Perhaps you could take up lawn bowling!"

8

SAMe Breakthrough

As yet, few folk know about **S-adenosylmethionine (SAMe)**. To biochemists, however, it ranks almost equal in importance with the primary energy molecule of the human body, adenosine triphosphate (ATP). SAMe works in just about every cell in your body as the active form of the essential amino acid methionine. It performs such a wide variety of functions, it would take this whole book to describe them. Here, we are concerned only with its benefit for joint disorders. And it's a biggie.

As I stated above, using glucosamine in conjunction with essential fats over the last decade, we have had a success rate of over 60% with both arthritis patients and athletes. In 1994, medical nutrition advocates, including the Colgan Institute, finally pushed through the Dietary Supplementation and Health Education Act (DSHEA), which allows all Americans free access to nutrient supplements. Many previously banned substances immediately became available. SAMe is one of them. Since then we have added SAMe to all our treatment protocols for arthritis, and inflammatory conditions of the joints and soft tissues, with a big increase in success.

We were interested in SAMe because studies with animals showed conclusively that intramuscular injections of SAMe increase both the number of chondrocytes in cartilage and the thickness of the cartilage pad.[1] Remember, the chondrocyte is the only living element in cartilage. It produces all the proteoglycans and collagen that make up the cartilage structure. Any nutrient that can increase the number of chondrocytes should be seized upon with glee. The big question to be answered was, does it work orally?

Oral SAMe Works

The answer came from more animal studies in the mid '80s which demonstrated easy intestinal absorption of oral SAMe and subsequent anti-inflammatory and analgesic actions.[2] Armed with this evidence, researchers throughout the world set to work. Extensive studies in Italy, with 22,000 arthritis patients over five years, showed without a doubt that SAMe increases proteoglycans production by chondrocytes in human cartilage, with no toxicity and virtually no side-effects.[3]

Most of these studies were done with patients classified as osteoarthritic. But SAMe also has beneficial effects on rheumatoid arthritis. One of the classic signs of rheumatoid conditions is the auto-immune attack on the joint and synovial membrane, especially by the potent immune component, **tumor necrosis factor** (TNF). In 1997, researchers in Spain published important results in the British Journal of Rheumatology, showing that SAMe restores synovial cells after they have been damaged by TNF. SAMe's specific inhibition of TNF damage suggests that using it to *prevent* auto-immune injury to the joints may be an even better way to go.[4]

SAMe Beats NSAIDs

Another great advantage of SAMe is that it reduces pain and loss of function sufficiently to enable patients to eliminate NSAIDs. Thus it helps enormously to set up the ideal conditions for joints to repair themselves. In a recent double-blind comparison at the famous Arthritis Clinic in Bad Abbach, Germany, patients diagnosed with osteoarthritis of the knees, hips and spine, were given either 1200 milligrams of SAMe or 1200 milligrams of **ibuprofen** daily for four weeks. Clinical results of the two treatments were equal for reduction of pain, swelling and stiffness, and for increased range of motion.[5]

A similar double-blind study compared 1200 milligrams of SAMe with the tolerable dose of 750 milligrams of **naproxyn** (Naprosyn). Both treatments had equal effects on pain, but the SAMe caused fewer side-effects and was judged the better treatment all round.[6]

The Auerbach Clinic in Bensheim, Germany, reports similar benefits of SAMe in another double-blind comparison with **indomethacin**.[7] SAMe is equal in anti-inflammatory and analgesic effects to common medical drugs, has no harsh side-effects and produces better compliance.

SAMe And Joint Regeneration

Another important finding comes from research on arthritis of the knee by Dr A Maccagno at Hospital Frances in Buenos Aires, Argentina. He showed not only that SAMe produced equal clinical results to the anti-inflammatory drug **piroxicam**, but also that patients given SAMe maintained the improvements in symptoms and in function for a considerable period after the SAMe was withdrawn. Improvements quickly faded after piroxicam was withdrawn. This continuation of benefits long after the SAMe treatment ended, adds clinical evidence to the biochemical evidence that SAMe helps to rebuild joints.[8]

The longest controlled study with SAMe continued for two years. Under the control of Dr B Konig at the University of Maintz, Germany, 10 physicians in various parts of Germany treated 108 patients diagnosed with chronic arthritis of knees, hips and spine. Patients received 600 milligrams of SAMe daily for four weeks, then only 400 milligrams per day for the rest of two years. Even with this small dosage, clinical improvements began within the first week and continued, in many cases progressively, for the whole two-year period.

Examination of the patients at six, 12, 18 and 24 months showed no further arthritic degeneration, indicating that SAMe was not only relieving pain and increasing range of motion, but was also preventing the progress of the disease. Most important, 18 patients showed total remission of symptoms — their long-term arthritis disappeared.[9]

SAMe For Fibromyalgia

Many cases of fibromyalgia and chronic fatigue syndrome are more properly classified as arthritis. So the potent analgesic and anti-inflammatory actions of SAMe on joint and soft tissues should work on these cases also. And they do. In a double-blind study at the University of Pisa in Italy, patients diagnosed with fibromyalgia were given SAMe or a placebo. SAMe significantly reduced the number of trigger points and tender areas.[10]

A more recent double-blind study by Dr S Jacobsen at Frederiksberg Hospital in Copenhagen, Denmark, confirms these findings. Fibromyalgia patients were given either 800 milligrams of SAMe or a placebo, daily for six weeks. By the last week, the SAMe patients showed big reductions in pain, fatigue and morning stiffness. Side effects — nil.[11]

Equally important, in these studies SAMe significantly improved the depression that often accompanies fibromyalgia, a mood-elevating effect, also noted frequently in studies of SAMe and osteoarthritis. I show you why in Chapters 9 and 10.

The research reviewed above is representative of the growing body of evidence that, even when used alone, SAMe offers great promise for treatment of numerous types of arthritis. In combination with essential fats and glucosamine sulfate, it is proving to be a real breakthrough.

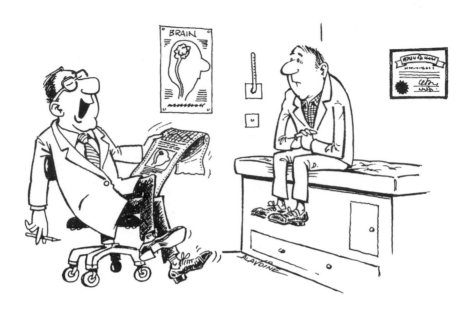

"I'm pleased to tell you, our new computerized analysis has finally worked out what's wrong with your head. You're basically stupid!"

9

The Homocysteine Connection

Rarely seen in the first half of this century, over the last 40 years elevated homocysteine in the blood has become a common condition, now affecting many millions of people in Western Society. As we will see, it is another telling example of human creation of disease through the destruction of essential nutrients in our food and the adoption of lifestyles that fail to provide sufficient amounts of the structural materials required to maintain the human body.

Most folk now know of Dr Kilmer McCully's research showing that elevated homocysteine is a strong risk factor for cardiovascular disease. In February 1998, in a guest editorial in the Journal of the American Medical Association, McCully recounts the long road he traveled to achieve medical acceptance.

The same issue of the journal details the research that vindicates his 30 years of patient work.[1,2] Little did he know, he was also pioneering the route to prevention and cure of arthritis.

Toxic effects of elevated homocysteine are not confined to the cardiovascular system. It also invades your brain, spinal cord and joints to promote a wide range of illnesses, including fibromyalgia, chronic fatigue, various forms of arthritis, depression and Alzheimer's disease.[3-7]

How Homocysteine Rises

We know from McCully's work, and from the research of hundreds of scientists who now collaborate with him, exactly which essential structural materials are missing from our diets, that allow homocysteine to rise. A quick peek at the chemistry reveals all. Homocysteine is a normal component of your body, an intermediate in the orchestrated symphony of biochemical events that keep you healthy. Folic acid and vitamin B_{12} (and probably vitamin B_6) act in concert to prevent homocysteine from rising to toxic levels by converting it back to the non-toxic essential amino acid **methionine**.[1-9] The cycle is shown in Figure 4.

This chemistry is intimately connected with SAMe. Remember from the last chapter how SAMe is the activated form of methionine used by almost every cell of your body in what are called **methylation reactions**. Well, if the body is short of folic acid and vitamin B_{12}, then a lot of your methionine gets tied up as elevated homocysteine, reducing the amount available for the body to maintain a normal level of SAMe.[1-9] Even a slight or intermittent deficiency of vitamin B_{12} and folic acid, if continued over years, allows homocysteine levels to gradually rise and

SAMe levels to gradually fall.[3-9]   SAMe probably works so well on arthritis precisely because arthritics are short of it.

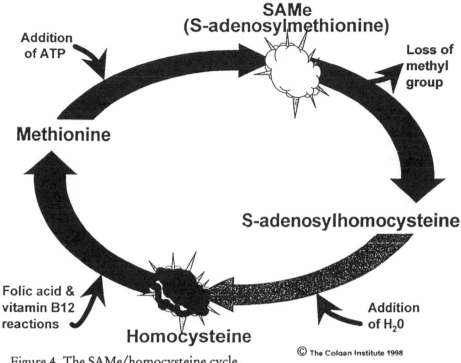

Figure 4. The SAMe/homocysteine cycle.

© The Colgan Institute 1998

Folic Acid & Vitamin B12 Deficiencies Rampant

If my analysis is correct, then folic acid and vitamin B_{12} deficiencies should be widespread in Western Society, and these deficiencies should be linked with high homocysteine levels. The latest review of studies of folic acid intake in Europe has just been completed by Dr A de Bree and colleagues at the Department of Human Nutrition of Wageningen University in

Holland. Mean dietary intake of folic acid is only 291 micrograms per day for men and 247 micrograms per day for women. This is woefully insufficient to prevent a toxic increase in homocysteine. As these researchers indicate, to keep homocysteine at healthy levels requires a *minimal* daily intake of 350 micrograms of folic acid.[10,11]

Similarly low folic acid intake is widespread in the US, where the folate content of a good diet is only 280 - 300 micrograms and the average daily intake is a lot less than that.[12] The folic acid intake in America has declined in concert with the degradation of our food, such that the previous RDA of 400 micrograms was reduced to 200 micrograms to suit. That's all you get in an average American diet. No surprise then that homocysteine levels are high and rising, despite continuing recommendations from various health authorities that the public should have a minimum folic acid intake of 400 micrograms per day.[3-9]

In Britain also, the latest National Diet and Nutrition Survey (1997) reports widespread, low intake of folic acid and vitamin B_{12}, strongly correlated with high homocysteine levels. Researchers there conclude that the link between homocysteine and vitamin deficiency is so strong, that plasma homocysteine can be used as a measure not only of folic acid status but also of vitamin B_{12} status in the British population.[13]

Leading researchers in Europe and America concur that high plasma homocysteine is a reliable marker of both folate and vitamin B_{12} deficiencies.[2,14] If you want to *prevent* certain illness, get these vitamins every day.

High Homocysteine/Low SAMe Damage Your Brain

The next step along our path to beat arthritis is to show that folic acid and vitamin B_{12} deficiencies, and consequent high homocysteine and low SAMe levels, cause mental degeneration and depression.

The latest review of studies of older people worldwide has just been completed at the Department of Clinical Medicine of Perugia University in Italy by Dr L Parnetti and colleagues. The data reveal that low intakes of folic acid and vitamin B_{12}, and consequent high homocysteine and low SAMe levels, are accompanied by depression and dementia.[4]

A similar review of the controlled studies of people of all ages was published in 1997 by Dr T Bottiglieri and group from the Institute of Metabolic Diseases of Baylor University Medical Center in Dallas, Texas. They found that folic acid and vitamin B_{12} deficiencies, and consequent elevated homocysteine, cause depression and dementia, and also damage the myelin sheaths that protect the nerves in your brain.[8]

High brain homocysteine also causes high production of **homocysteic acid** in the brain, known to cause excessive brain stimulation and cognitive disturbance.[4] Worse, high brain homocysteine causes **microangiopathy** (micro-strokes) damaging small blood vessels with resulting permanent mental impairment.[15]

High Homocysteine/Low SAMe In Alzheimer's

Alzheimer's disease provides further evidence that high levels of homocysteine are linked with brain damage. Alzheimer's patients tested at University hospitals in Leuven, Belgium and Munster, Germany, showed more frequent deficiencies of folic acid and vitamin B_{12}, and higher levels of homocysteine than mentally healthy controls.[7]

In another recent study, Dr L Morrison and colleagues of the University of Toronto in Ontario, Canada, measured SAMe in Alzheimer's. Every one of the Alzheimer's patients had very low SAMe levels — only 15 - 33% of the levels of healthy controls. Yet in Parkinson's disease, which is a different type of brain degeneration, SAMe levels are often normal. These findings indicate that low SAMe is not simply a consequence of general brain degeneration, but *is an active cause* of the depression and severe memory loss that are markers of Alzheimer's.[16]

Studies reviewed in this chapter show that the low folate and vitamin B_{12} intake endemic in Western Society, damage both joints and brain by allowing homocysteine to rise to pathological levels. Folk using the drug methotrexate to treat their arthritis should be especially warned, because methotrexate interferes with folate metabolism and worsens the problem.[17] Chapter 10 shows you how to solve it.

10

Beating Arthritic Depression

The discovery that low folic acid and low vitamin B_{12} cause high homocysteine and low SAMe is vital to our understanding of fibromyalgia, chronic fatigue, and both rheumatoid and osteo forms of arthritis. As we saw in Chapter 9, this syndrome is directly toxic to your joints and brain. Arthritic disorders are frequently accompanied by chronic depression and cognitive disturbance, which used to be explained away as psychological reactions to the unremitting discomfort. The evidence now indicates that arthritic depression results from direct poisoning of the brain.

The depression and other mental symptoms of arthritis patients are usually treated with a wide variety of toxic anti-depressant drugs that have no place in the human body, and side effects often cause more harm than the blahs they alleviate. Also, these drugs do nothing to treat the poisoning of the brain that caused the depression in the first place. So, if it can be treated and prevented by non-toxic natural substances that also heal the joints, we should jump at the chance.

I have room to cite only a fraction of the pile of studies sitting on my desk. These are all recent discoveries published from late 1996 to 1998, so you cannot blame physicians if they are unaware of the new developments. The time lag between scientific discovery and adoption into medical practice is huge — *seven to fourteen years*. The following are a few representative papers from universities all over the world that show you just how the evidence is stacking up.

Homocysteine in Arthritis

The latest study of homocysteine and rheumatoid arthritis is by Dr R Roubenoff and colleagues at Tufts University in Boston, Massachusetts. They report that nearly half of all rheumatoid patients tested showed folic acid deficiency, and a high proportion showed vitamin B_{12} deficiency. *All* the patients showed elevated homocysteine. Their blood homocysteine levels were 33% higher than healthy hospital workers used as controls.[1]

With fibromyalgia and chronic fatigue, a new study of women patients has just been published by Dr B Regland and team at the Institute of Clinical Neuroscience of Göteborg University in Sweden. They found that *every one* of these women had elevated homocysteine levels in their cerebrospinal fluid.[2]

Many recent studies show unequivocally that fibromyalgia, chronic fatigue, rheumatoid arthritis and osteoarthritis are all accompanied by a very high incidence of chronic depression. [1-7] The new evidence linking depression in arthritis with the syndrome of folic acid/vitamin B_{12} deficiency and consequent high homocysteine/low SAMe levels, indicates strongly that correction of this relatively simple problem could not only relieve arthritis, but may also eliminate its attendant mood disorders.

Folate, B₁₂ and SAMe Reduce Homocysteine

The next step on our path to beat the depression and pain of arthritis is to examine whether vitamins can reduce homocysteine levels, and whether SAMe is a useful addition to this treatment. In 1997, Dr M Ward and team at the University of Ulster in Ireland, confirmed earlier work on folate supplementation. They show unequivocally that 400 micrograms per day of folic acid reliably reduces homocysteine levels.[8]

The latest study, published in the New England Journal of Medicine in April 1998 by Dr M Malinow and colleagues, gave patients with coronary artery disease a breakfast cereal fortified with folic acid. Fortification with 499 micrograms and 655 micrograms of folic acid per day raised plasma folic acid by 65% and 106% respectively, and reduced homocysteine levels by 11% and 14%.[9] From this and similar studies, the Colgan Institute has derived a dose of 800 micrograms – 3.0 milligrams per day of folic acid as appropriate for arthritis patients.

After reviewing 35 recent studies, Dr M Moghadasian and colleagues at St Paul's Hospital in Vancouver, Canada, recommend that vitamin B_{12} and folic acid be used together to lower homocysteine levels.[10] It's sensible to always include vitamin B_{12} in a supplementation regimen for two reasons. First, as we saw in Chapter 9, vitamin B_{12} is required for the SAMe/homocysteine cycle. Second, many folk, especially older folk, have a vitamin B_{12} deficiency which would be masked by folic acid supplementation alone, and would continue to progressively damage the brain.[11] From all controlled studies to date, the Colgan Institute has derived a dose of vitamin B_{12} of 100 – 400 micrograms per day as both safe and effective.

SAMe works too. A new study has just been published by Dr F Loehrer and colleagues at University Children's Hospital in Basel, Switzerland. They show that, even in healthy subjects, 400 milligrams of SAMe per day improves folic acid metabolism and reduces homocysteine levels.[12] At the Colgan Institute, we use a minimum of 400 milligrams of SAMe per day with arthritis patients.

SAMe Against Depression

Folic acid, vitamin B_{12} and SAMe all work to correct the chemical imbalance that seems to be the main cause of depression in arthritis. But it is SAMe that is proving most effective. A review of SAMe and mood disorders by Dr R Baldessarini at Harvard Medical School, Boston, indicates that SAMe supplementation relieves depression in both psychiatric patients and other patients.[13] Studies also show that SAMe improves cognition and reduces depression in some cases of Alzheimer's.[14]

SAMe also reduces depression in numerous forms of arthritis. In a two-year study of osteoarthritics, Dr B Konig and colleagues at the University of Pisa in Italy, report that 400 milligrams of SAMe per day caused a big improvement in mood.[15]

In a placebo-controlled study of fibromyalgia at the same university, Dr A Tavoni and team reported a high incidence of depression. SAMe supplementation provided effective relief.[16]

In another controlled study of fibromyalgia, Dr S Jacobsen of the Department of Rheumatology of Fredericksburg Hospital in Copenhagen, Denmark, measured emotional states before and after six weeks of SAMe treatment. Compared with a placebo group, the patients given SAMe showed significant improvement.[17]

From these many similar studies, the message for sufferers from all forms of arthritis and its accompanying depression is loud and clear — folic acid and vitamin B_{12} deficiencies are rampant in Western Society. These deficiencies lead to high levels of homocysteine and low levels of SAMe. This syndrome creates a double-whammy toxic condition for your joints and your brain, a condition that promotes both arthritis and depression.

Supplementation with non-toxic amounts of folic acid and vitamin B_{12} reduces homocysteine and increases SAMe, thereby restoring metabolism of these substances towards normal healthy levels. Additional supplementation with non-toxic amounts of SAMe enhances this simple strategy, helping to heal your brain and your joints by providing the essential structural materials they require for normal function. If you have arthritis — don't leave home without them.

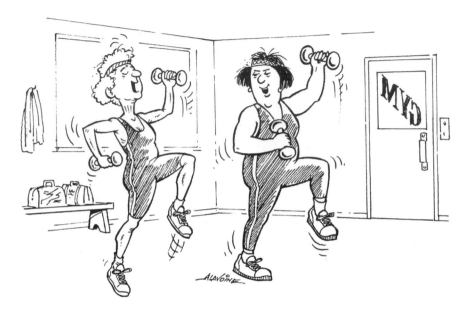

"I have the body
of a 20 year old!"

"Well, you'd better give it back,
...you're getting it all wrinkled!"

11

Antioxidants Against Arthritis

In 1956, Dr Denman Harmon at the University of Nebraska first proposed that humans grow old and diseased primarily because of **uncontrolled oxidation.** His short, three-page paper in the journal Gerontology, changed forever our conception of the degenerative diseases of aging.[1]   Now, over 40 years later, thousands of studies worldwide have confirmed that he is right.[2] As I document in my book, **The New Nutrition,** cardiovascular disease, many forms of cancer, diabetes, cataracts, macular degeneration, multiple different infections, and burns and other wounds all cause their long-term damage by uncontrolled oxidation.[3]

This is not surprising because uncontrolled oxidation is the most pervasive process of decay on Earth. The rusting of steel, the browning of a cut apple, the rotting of meat and the aging of human flesh all occur by uncontrolled oxidation. Ultra-violet light, many pesticides, poisons, air pollutants, even nuclear radiation do their damage mainly by uncontrolled oxidation.[2]

It's tough to beat. One year after completion of the New Statue of Liberty, its copper surface protected by the most advanced methods known to science, the American Institute of Architects had to report to Congress that it was being eaten away by the highly oxidative air pollution of New York. Eventually even glass and granite rock oxidize to dust.

Free Radical Damage

In a very small nutshell, it happens like this. Each atom of stable matter has pairs of electrons spinning around its nucleus. Electrons spin in pairs to balance their electromagnetic forces. As long as these forces are balanced, the atom, be it of rock or human flesh, spins merrily along, forever as far as we know, and does not interfere with its neighbors.

But if an atom loses an electron, it becomes a **free radical** — an atom gone mad, with a crazily spinning unpaired electron that grabs at every nearby atom with its unbalanced electromagnetic force. Acting much like a strong magnet, it tears an electron out of the nearest intact atom of flesh. Or it can lose the battle and surrender its crazy electron to the nearest atom of flesh. Either way, this process creates a second free radical which then goes on to create a third and a fourth. Within seconds you have a chain reaction of free radical damage.

The very act of breathing produces millions of oxygen free radicals that would kill you outright were it not for the miraculous design of the human body. Your body comes equipped with endogenous antioxidants, mainly **catalase, superoxide dismutase** and **glutathione** which, in combination with nutrient antioxidants from food, disarm many of these nasties.

But, you cannot disarm enough of them to stop disease and degeneration. Especially in modern society, where we have increased our oxidation burden manyfold, with air pollutants, water pollutants, man-made pesticides, herbicides, drugs and a plethora of toxic artificial chemicals now inextricably embedded in our food chain. To keep these villains at bay you need the help of the new antioxidant science.

Antioxidants To The Rescue

Exogenous antioxidants are special nutrient molecules which can give up an electron or receive an extra electron without themselves becoming very damaging radicals. They do become radicals, but other antioxidants immediately step in to disarm them further, until step-by-step the original free radicals are reduced to harmless carbon dioxide, which you breathe out, and water, which the body can re-use.

Astute readers will realize from even my brief sketch of oxidation damage, that having a good supply of antioxidants in your body is one of the best insurance policies against disease. You will realize also that antioxidants operate only as a team, each one backing up the others in the step-by-step reduction of free radicals to harmless waste. Consequently, taking any one or two or three antioxidants, as is often advised in the popular health literature, is unwise. Such a strategy leaves free radicals only partly neutralized and may *increase* the uncontrolled oxidative stress on your body. You need a full mix.

My recent book, **Antioxidants: The Real Story,** documents the main types of free radicals, and the types and amounts of nutrient antioxidants you need to combat them. Here I have room only to reproduce the essentials of the table from that book.[4] The mixed antioxidant supplement you need is detailed in Table 2. Sources and brands are given in Chapter 13.

Some physicians still have lingering doubts about long-term use of nutrient antioxidants. These doubts are eagerly seized and blown out of proportion by media hacks who know that bad news outsells good.

To counteract such misinformation, I record in my books the public statements of many eminent scientists, who have seen the evidence on antioxidants grow so convincing that they have publicly endorsed them. Even the famous Dr Kenneth Cooper, who pooh-poohed antioxidants when I first approached him about them in the early '80s, has now written his own book extolling their virtues.[5] And in 1994, Dr Jeffrey Blumberg, one of America's top government researchers at the USDA Human Nutrition Research Center, recommended publicly that everyone take antioxidants. He concluded:

> **We have the confidence that these things really do work.[6]**

Table 2. Daily Antioxidant Mix to Combat Arthritis

Antioxidant Nutrient ‡	Daily Amount		
Vitamin E (IU)** (D-alpha-tocopherol succinate)‡	800	–	1200
Vitamin C (gm) (Ascorbic Acid, mixed mineral ascorbates, ascorbyl palmitate)	2.0	–	5.0
Beta-carotene (IU)**	15,000	–	30,000
Coenzyme Q10 (g)	15	–	30
L-glutathione (mg)	100	–	150
N-acetyl cysteine (mg) ♯	100	–	175
Selenium (mcg) (L-selenomethionine)	200	–	300
Iron (mg) (Iron picolinate)	10	–	14
Zinc (mg) (Zinc picolinate)	15	–	25
Copper (mg) (Copper gluconate)	0.5	–	1.25
Manganese (mg) (Manganese gluconate)	2.0	–	4.0
Alpha-lipoic acid (mg)	100	–	200
Lycopene (mg)	50	–	100
Lutein (mg)	6	–	9
Rutin, hesperidin, naringin (mg) (mixed citrus flavonoids)	200	–	300
Procyanidins (mg) (grape seed extract, standardized to 95%)	150	–	200
Catechins (mg) (green tea extracts standardized to 20%)	20	–	40
Bilobetin, amentoflavones (mg) (ginkgo biloba extract standardized to 24%)	8	–	12
Silymarin, taxifolin (mg) (milk thistle extract standardized to 80%)	50	–	100
Genestein, diadzein (mg) (soybean extract standardized to 10%)	10	–	20
Anthocyanins (mg) (bilberry extract standardized to 25%)	10	–	15
Melatonin (mg)	1.0	–	1.75
S-adenosylmethionine (mg)	400	–	800

** IU, International Units are obsolete measures no longer used in science. But because they continue to appear on supplement labels, they are used here for convenience.

‡ Preferred forms of nutrients used by the Colgan Institute are given, because different forms of the same nutrient have widely different absorption rates and degrees of efficacy. The figures cannot be applied to other forms.

♯ N-acetyl cysteine should be used only in conjunction with at least three times the amount of vitamin C. Otherwise n-acetyl cysteine can precipitate as cysteine in the kidneys and possibly cause kidney stones in sensitive individuals.

The latest endorsement of antioxidants comes from Dr Ranjit Chandra, in an editorial in the Journal of the American Medical Association, May 7, 1997, endorsing the effects of vitamin C and vitamin E against arterial damage. An eminent doctor, speaking to doctors in their leading medical journal, he states:

> **The era of nutrient supplements to support health and reduce illness is here to stay.**[7]

Arthritics Short On Antioxidants

Despite these recommendations from leading medical authorities, the diets of many folk suffering from arthritis are low in antioxidants. In a representative study, Dr J M Kremer and J Bigaouette at the Department of Medicine of Albany Medical College, New York, examined the diets of rheumatoid arthritis patients. As we might expect from Chapter 9, they found that patients were low in the non-antioxidant, folic acid. But they were also low in the important antioxidant minerals — zinc and copper. The researchers concluded that rheumatoid patients should take regular multi-vitamin/mineral supplements.[8]

In another recent study, Dr J Stone and colleagues at the Department of Rheumatology at Waikato Hospital in Hamilton, New Zealand, also examined the diets of rheumatoid arthritic patients. Less than half the patients got even the low Recommended Daily Intake (RDI) of folic acid (200 mcg). But, more important for antioxidant status, less than one-third of patients ate the RDI for vitamin E. Only 10% ate the RDI for zinc and only 6% ate the RDI for selenium.[9]

The deficiency of selenium in arthritis was confirmed in a new study by Dr K Heinle and colleagues at Ludwig-Maximillian University in Munchen, Germany. They found that blood levels of selenium in patients with rheumatoid arthritis, were 30% lower than in healthy controls.[10]

Another representative study has just been published by Dr M Sklodowska and team in the prestigious journal, **Clinical and Experimental Rheumatology**. They showed that, compared with healthy controls, children with juvenile rheumatoid arthritis had high levels of free radicals in their bodies and low levels of vitamin E in their plasma.[11]

These studies are just the tip of the iceberg of emerging evidence that folk with arthritis, especially in its many rheumatoid forms, have low levels of antioxidants in their bodies. Consequently, they are likely to have high levels of uncontrolled oxidation. Does this oxidation cause arthritic degeneration? You bet!

Arthritic Damage From Oxidation

Vital research showing that uncontrolled oxidation is a major villain in joint and associated soft tissue diseases, is flooding into medical journals from laboratories worldwide. It is all new discovery. In a representative study in 1995, at London Hospital Medical College in England, Dr C J Morris and colleagues showed that uncontrolled oxidation causes joint inflammation.[12]

In another typical example in 1996, at the Medical University in Iasi, Romania, Dr R Chiriac and team showed that inflammatory conditions of various forms of rheumatoid arthritis are caused by oxygen free radicals.[13]

In 1997, Dr G W Comstock and colleagues at Johns Hopkins University in Baltimore, examined the development of rheumatoid arthritis and lupus erythematosus. They studied folk whose antioxidant status had been measured as much as 15 years *before* they showed any signs of disease. The results are explicit. Subjects whose antioxidant intake was high did not develop arthritis. Those who did develop rheumatoid arthritis or lupus had low intakes of vitamin A, beta-carotene and vitamin E. In short, antioxidant intake predicted the development of arthritis up to 15 years later. The researchers concluded that low antioxidant status is a risk factor for arthritis.[14]

Antioxidants Curb Arthritis

Do supplementary antioxidants help once you have arthritis? Yes they do. In a new study from Ludwig-Maximillian University in Germany, a group of rheumatoid arthritis patients were divided in half and given either 200 micrograms of selenium per day or a placebo, as an addition to their normal treatment. After three months, the placebo subjects showed little improvement. But the subjects receiving selenium showed significantly reduced inflammation, plus large reductions in pain, swelling and morning stiffness.[10] Even supplementation with this single antioxidant alone was beneficial.

Antioxidants also help osteoarthritis. In a typical study, Dr. T McAlindon and colleagues at the Arthritis Center of Boston University, Massachusetts examined osteoarthritis of the knees. They used subjects from the famous "Framingham Osteoarthritis Cohort Study" who had complete knee examinations between 1983 – 1985 and again between 1992 – 1993. They found that high intakes of vitamin C reduced the risk of cartilage loss by 300%![15] Most important, even in subjects with confirmed chronic knee osteoarthritis, they found that high intakes of vitamin C reduced the progression of cartilage damage.[15]

These and similar studies indicate that folk who have lupus, rheumatoid arthritis or osteoarthritis, should take mixed antioxidants every day. There are no studies yet on arthritic fibromyalgia and chronic fatigue. But I'll bet my new boots it will turn out the same for them.

Before you start, remember that this treatment, though non-toxic, is still experimental. At the Colgan Institute, we undertake the nutritional treatment of arthritis only in collaboration with the patient's physician. You should take this book and the medical references to your physician. It is the physician's job, not mine, to decide whether this treatment is right for your particular case.

SAMe Is An Antioxidant

For folk with arthritis, SAMe is a bonus addition to the antioxidant list. New research shows that SAMe has antioxidant properties that are a boon to joints. Dr J P De la Cruz and team at the School of Medicine of the University of Malaga in Spain, discovered in October 1997 that SAMe supplementation increases the vital endogenous antioxidant glutathione.[16]

Another 1997 study by Dr P J Evans and colleagues at Kings College, London University in England, confirmed that SAMe acts as a precursor for glutathione. Equally important, they showed that SAMe itself directly neutralizes one of the most toxic free radicals, **the hydroxyl radical**, and also inhibits hydroxyl radical production.[17]

Even if you do nothing else, persuade your physician that you should take your antioxidants and your SAMe every day. I hope, however, that I have convinced you to do a bit more than that to beat the curse of arthritis. If you are keen to banish it from your life forever, the full program given in Chapter 13 is tailor-made for the job.

> *Be kind to your knees,*
> *You'll miss them when they're gone*

12

The Hormone Solution

Hormones can cause — or prevent — arthritis. No doubt about it. But the research is still young and spirited, galloping wildly in many directions, often confusing motion with progress. So I hope you will forgive me if my analysis is sharp, uncompromising, aiming to cut to the nub.

From questions I get at lectures, it's clear that many folk are only vaguely aware that female bodies make and need what used to be called "male" hormones, such as testosterone. Similarly, male bodies make and need what used to be called "female" hormones, such as estrogen. For example, as documented in my book, **Hormonal Health,** both male and female brains require a constant supply of estrogen for normal function, and both male and female libidos run on testosterone.[1] Understanding the various gender roles of all the hormones is essential to work out the effects of hormones on arthritis.

Whenever I lecture to a women's organization, most of the audience agrees with me that female bodies are hormonally disadvantaged. With menopause, women lose their **estrogen**, their **progesterone**, most of their **testosterone** and most of their **dehydroepiandrosterone (DHEA)**. The DHEA is first to go, starting a sharp decline during perimenopause, age 40 – 45.[1] Along with it the brain hormone **melatonin**, the synchronizer of the whole hormone cascade in your body, also shows a sharp decline.[1] All five of these hormones decline with age and are highly correlated with the incidence of arthritis.

In women, the various forms of rheumatoid arthritis increase rapidly in incidence between ages 35 and 50. Overall, rheumatoid arthritis attacks at least *three* times as many women as men. At menopause, incidence of the various forms of osteoarthritis also rises dramatically. Overall, after age 45, osteoarthritis affects *ten* times as many women as men.[2,3]

Some doom merchants claim that these correlations are merely coincidence, that the female body loses its hormones about the age it is degenerating into arthritis anyway, and the hormones have little to do with the inevitable decay of joints. They are dead wrong.

Estrogen Against Rheumatoid Arthritis

Let's look first at rheumatoid arthritis. In addition to the links between these disorders and menopause, four lines of evidence show that the hormonal loss at menopause is a direct cause of the higher incidence of arthritis in women.

First, in contrast to women, men rarely develop rheumatoid arthritis until age 45. Thereafter, male incidence of rheumatoid arthritis rises in concert with their gradual loss of DHEA and testosterone (the male's main source of estrogen) into old age.[1-3]

Second, research on young women shows that rheumatoid arthritis fluctuates in concert with the hormonal changes during menstruation, pregnancy and post-partum.[4] In addition, new research shows that young women with rheumatoid arthritis also have severe hormone deficits. In a recent representative study, Dr F Flaisler and colleagues at the Carmeau Hospital in Nimes, France, evaluated ovarian function in young women with rheumatoid arthritis. They used only women who were not on contraceptive pills because, as I have shown elsewhere, these drugs disrupt normal hormone function with disastrous side-effects.[1] Flaisler found that all the women had very low levels of estrogen, so low that many of them were unable to become pregnant.[4]

The third line of evidence linking low estrogen with rheumatoid conditions, concerns new discoveries of specific estrogenic effects on immunity. Low levels of estrogen allow a particular part of your immune system, called **Th1 cellular immunity**, to run wild. Increased Th1 activity is now established as a major promoter of rheumatoid arthritis.[3]

Estrogen And Bone Loss

Low levels of estrogen also cause rapid bone loss. Dr Robert Lindsay of Columbia University has documented this problem meticulously for the last 25 years. The average post-menopausal loss of bone is shown in Figure 5. Unless women use hormone replacement (we'll look at the *right kind* of hormone replacement below), about a quarter of their bone mass disappears by age 65.[5]

What has bone loss got to do with rheumatoid arthritis? A whole lot. Bone decalcification is a big part of the disease, especially in the big thigh bone, the femur, where it sockets into your hip. Rheumatoid arthritis patients have double the usual risk of a hip fracture.[6]

Recent research also shows that the higher a woman's bone mass, the less chance she has of developing rheumatoid arthritis. Even if she has a rheumatoid condition, estrogen replacement and consequent increased bone mass relieves the disease considerably, though it does not cure it.[6]

Estrogen In Osteoarthritis

Bone loss is also critical for osteoarthritis, much of which involves destruction of the ends of the bones. Here the evidence in favor of hormone replacement is very strong. In a new, carefully-controlled study, Dr S A Oliveria at the Department of Epidemiology of Harvard School of Public Health, reports that past use or current use of estrogen replacement reduces the risk of osteoarthritis of hand, hip and knee.[7]

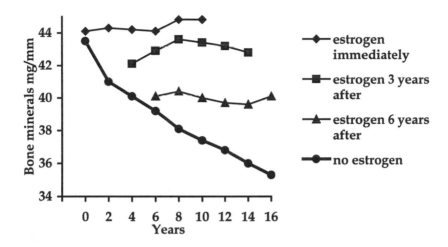

Figure 5. Long-term prevention of bone loss by estrogen. The earlier estrogen is begun after loss of ovarian function, the greater the bone mass retained. (Source: Lindsay & Cosman, see reference 5)

Dr T D Spector and colleagues at St Thomas's Hospital in London, have also confirmed that current users of hormone replacement receive a big protective effect against osteoarthritis of the hand and knee.[8]

In other supporting research, Dr M C Nevitt and colleagues at the University of California, San Francisco, studied 4366 women, aged 65 and over, enrolled in a study on hip fractures. Women currently using estrogen replacement had a greatly reduced risk of *any* osteoarthritis, especially of the hip. Users of hormone replacement for 10 years or more had the greatest chance of avoiding the disease.[9]

Another new study from Sweden confirms these findings. Women using hormone replacement, who keep their bodyweight under control, have little need for hip replacement.[10] These studies are all representative of the emerging evidence that a low level of estrogen in your body is an open invitation to arthritis.

Estrogen Supports Collagen

The protective effect of estrogen replacement in preventing bone loss is shown in Figure 5. Not yet so well known is estrogen's protection of **collagen**, the main protein in your body that gives structure and form to your flesh. Loss of bodily collagen in women rises sharply with menopause. First, the most estrogen-sensitive bodyparts, the reproductive organs, begin to lose structure and shrink in upon themselves. Then, though fat may hide it somewhat, facial flesh declines. Cheeks sag, lips thin and wrinkle, and eyes sink into their sockets as they lose supportive collagen.[1]

Medical scientists have known these facts for two decades,[11] but little if anything has been done to help women overcome what health authorities derisively call a "cosmetic problem." If they get anything at all, most women still receive the obsolete hormone replacement therapy of forty years ago.[1] With strong evidence that estrogen protects the heart, bones, brain, flesh, and now the joints,[1,12] we are on the happy verge of a hormonal revolution.

Numerous recent studies show that estrogen replacement reduces and even reverses the loss of flesh caused by hormone decline at menopause. It does so largely by restoring collagen.[13,14]

In 1993, for example, the Chelsea and Westminster Hospital in London, gave post-menopausal women estrogen to prevent osteoporosis. To their amazement, researchers found an increase in collagen throughout the body.[15] A 1994 study at St Francis of Assisi Hospital in Quebec confirmed these findings. Women given estrogen for 12 months had dramatic increases in collagen structures below the skin. They also experienced facial rejuvenation that gave them a whole new outlook on life.[16]

An additional aid to collagen that we add to estrogen comes from **procyanidins,** the flavonoids that give the dark blue color to black grapes, black cherries and blueberries. Though they do not rebuild collagen, procyanidins protect it from destruction.[17]

As we saw in earlier chapters, the two structural components of your joint cartilage are proteoglycans and collagen fibrils. If either one goes, so does the cartilage. Consequently, the new evidence that estrogen replacement rebuilds women's collagen suggests it may also protect against osteoarthritis by helping to rebuild cartilage. No studies yet exist that examine this potential benefit, but if researchers don't find it when they start looking, I'll eat my fishing hat.

Estrogen, DHEA Against Depression

Deficits of many bodily biochemicals can cause depression and other cognitive disorders. We have already seen the depression that occurs with the common deficiencies of folic acid, vitamin B_{12} and SAMe. Now we have to add estrogen and testosterone deficiencies to the list.

From perimenopause through menopause, rates of depression in women escalate dramatically.[1] Estrogen decline in menopause and its connection with depression is well accepted, but only recently have long-term studies shown that a woman's testosterone declines also.[18,19]   Leading many other researchers worldwide, Dr Barbara Sherwin of McGill University in Montreal has shown repeatedly that estrogen replacement reduces depression. When a little testosterone is added to the mix, many cases of depression disappear entirely.[20]

Fortunately, women don't have to take testosterone itself, a hazardous strategy at best.[1] DHEA will do the job nicely. DHEA is readily converted to testosterone in the female body.[1] In addition, DHEA levels are abnormally low in young women with rheumatoid arthritis, further evidence that this intermediate hormone is involved in the hormone cascade that helps prevent arthritis.[21]

You don't need a lot of DHEA. A small dose of 25 milligrams per day is sufficient to restore DHEA levels and to raise testosterone in most post-menopausal women.[1] A similar dose also works in men, not by raising male testosterone levels, but by supporting the whole system by which the male body produces testosterone and other steroid hormones.[1]

It will take a decade or more before these new discoveries are incorporated into medicine. Meanwhile with the right estrogen replacement, plus 25 milligrams of DHEA per day, a menopausal woman can defend both her brain and her emotions. I cover all the details in **Hormonal Health**.[1] You should take that book along with this one, plus the medical references to your physician, so that he or she can decide if such a treatment is right for you.

Progesterone Against Arthritis

Estrogen replacement does nothing to replace the progesterone that declines along with it during menopause. The dangers of replacing one hormone and not its companion and controller are now well known, the most prominent being increased risk of endometrial cancer.[1] Not yet well known is the effect of progesterone loss on arthritis. Women who use the usual estrogen replacement, without progesterone, still have a reduced risk of rheumatoid arthritis. However, they can develop a much increased risk of lupus.[2,22] This is an important discovery, because the various forms of the auto-immune disease lupus affect *fifteen* times as many women as men.[2,3]

"Whoa!" say some of my medical colleagues. Hormone replacement therapy today almost always includes progesterone, so women should be protected against lupus. They are misinformed. Usual hormone replacement does *not* include progesterone but rather **progestins,** man-made chemicals that may offer little protection against lupus.[1]

I document the many problems with progestins in **Hormonal Health**. In contrast, real progesterone has specific effects in controlling estrogen, and in suppressing immune reactions that may promote lupus. Real progesterone also helps to keep Th1 immunity under control, thereby further reducing the risk of rheumatoid arthritis.[3]

Hormone Replacement: The Right Stuff

Many women are wary of the usual hormone replacement prescribed today — and rightly so. My book **Hormonal Health** documents these problems in detail. The therapies it proposes are not yet accepted in official medical policies. Since publication three years ago, however, the solutions offered in **Hormonal Health** have been adopted by hundreds of physicians worldwide.

Briefly, usual hormone replacement utilizes the wrong forms of estrogen in too large a dose, together with synthetic progestins that do not control it properly. Women are rarely given the other hormones, specifically melatonin and DHEA, that the body also requires to balance the estrogen replacement.

Our Hormonal Health Program includes the correct forms of estrogen. We recommend the **Tri-Est** brand, which you can have dispensed by mail on your normal physician's prescription from the Women's International Pharmacy in Madison, Wisconsin at 1-800-279-5708.

We also recommend real progesterone, which can be obtained by prescription from the same source, either as a pill or as a cream to be rubbed into face and body. Don't be fooled, however, by all the false wild yam and other herbal creams claiming to contain progesterone. Our monthly magazine, the **Colgan Chronicles** (available from 1-800-668-2775), documents those creams on the market that contain real progesterone in any significant amount.

Remember, before you even think of trying any of these therapies, consult your physician. Hormones are not innocuous. Don't mess with them without the right professional help.

Individual biochemistry varies so greatly that only your health professional has the intimate knowledge of your case necessary to make the decision that such therapy may be right for you.

Nutritional Effects on Hormones

The recently discovered effects of nutrient deficiencies, especially mineral deficiencies, on hormones are so numerous it would take this whole book to cover them. The best I can do here is to give some examples of common nutrients that are deficient in America. Chromium deficiency, which is present in the majority of Americans today[1] affects body levels of DHEA. Boron deficiency reduces estrogen and testosterone levels while boron supplementation increases them.[23] Potassium deficiency reduces testosterone levels and potassium supplementation increases them.[24] Zinc affects both testosterone and estrogen.[25]

A final example is the widespread essential fat deficiencies we discussed earlier. As well as all the other problems caused by insufficient essential fats, they also reduce the bioavailability of bodily estrogen, thereby promoting both arthritis and brain disorders.[26]

If you don't get a full complement of these and other essential nutrients every day, your hormones decline and your risk of arthritis increases. I cover the whole list of essential nutrients elsewhere.[1] The best way to ensure that you get yours is to take a complete multi-vitamin/mineral supplement every day. The best brands are Colgan Institute MC8, USANA Essentials, Twinlab and Solgar.

Herbal Alternatives To Hormones

Traditional herbals that affect hormone levels are gaining new popularity as alternatives to hormones, especially for treatment of menopausal symptoms. These plants appeal to the considerable number of women who are against hormones of any kind. Most used are red clover, Chinese angelica, licorice, chasteberry, black cohosh, soy isoflavones and strawberries for their boron. Only three, however, have any controlled trials that support their use. They are, black cohosh, chasteberry and soy isoflavones.

A standardized extract of black cohosh (*Cimicifuga racemosa*) is medically approved for treatment of menopause in Europe. The most prominent brand is **Remifemin**. Current evidence shows that this herb dramatically reduces sleep disorders, hot flashes and other symptoms of menopause. It achieves these effects primarily from estrogen-like compounds that bind to estrogen receptors and may pinch-hit for the hormone. Black cohosh also contains compounds that suppress output of luteinizing hormone.[27] There is no evidence, however, that the herb protects bones, joints or brain from long-term effects of the loss of estrogen or other hormones with menopause.

Chasteberry (*Vitex agnus castus*) is widely used in Europe as a treatment for menopausal symptoms and for menstrual problems. It contains a compound which increases the activity of dopamine, a prominent neurotransmitter in the brain that, among other functions, inhibits prolactin secretion.[28] In **Hormonal Health,** I cover many more ways to maintain dopamine activity, which declines with usual aging.[1] As with black cohosh, however, there is yet no evidence that chasteberry can protect your brain, bones or joints. A lot of research remains to be done on these herbs before I would recommend them as alternatives to hormone replacement.

Soy isoflavones, notably **genestein** and **diadzein** have weak but reliable estrogenic effects that can reduce or eliminate many symptoms of menopause.[29,30]   Recent research shows that soy isoflavones also reduce the risk of reproductive system cancers[31] and protect the cardiovascular system in older women.[32]   These widespread beneficial effects on multiple bodily systems indicate that soy isoflavones could be beneficial to joints also.   Though no studies have yet been done, the Colgan Institute analysis of the interactive chemistry of soy and estrogen, supports isoflavone use as an aid to healthy joints.   They are most easily obtained from traditionally made organic tofu and miso, though several brands of soy isoflavone supplements have appeared recently in the marketplace.   Best are Colgan Institute and Life Extension Foundation.

A particularly good supplement for joints is the combination of ion-exchange whey protein concentrate and soy protein with a high isoflavone content.

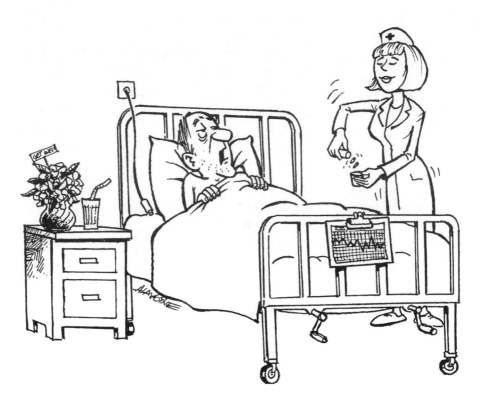

*"Are you sure those pills will kill the bacteria.
I don't want anything that will just make them mad!"*

13

The Road To Happy Joints

The first step to beat arthritis is to get your diet and your body lean and clean. I have not said much about the lean bit, because it is more than obvious how the constant weight of excess bodyfat aggravates arthritis. I give a comprehensive program to lose bodyfat in my book **The New Nutrition**.[1] Those who have tried numerous diets and weight-loss schemes on their own without success should join the Lean Team of the USANA company. The Lean Team Program, for which I was the design consultant, is a first-class, team-supported strategy for keeping bodyfat at bay lifelong. Running now for three years, it is the only program I know that has hard evidence of long-term success with the seriously overweight.

If you are not badly overweight, then the food and activity program given in this book will take care of it. You can review all the dietary details in Chapter 2. Here I will just summarize in a somewhat dotty ditty, which nevertheless helps folk to remember.

The Road To Happy Joints

To keep thine hand and back and eye
Free from the rheum that twists thy limb,
Eat spelt and barley corn and rye,
Fresh from the mill, ne'er stale from the bin,
And carrots, kale and pumpkins three
Quick from the garden into thee.
Take apples, pears, and peaches pie
And berries all when their season be.
Take fish from the sea and flowing stream,
Ne'er from salter nor pond, they've lost their glim.
Leave cows on the hill and pigs in the sty,
Else thou get the gout and rheumy eye.
Red wine and porter, ale and sack,
All put a burden on thy back.
Drink from the stream, fill thy cup to the rim.
Stay spare of belly and out of strife
Run from apothecary and surgeon's knife
And freedom of limb will bless thy life.

Michael Colgan

Getting Your Omega-3's

The next step after fixing your diet is to set the scene for joint repair. Omega-3 and omega-6 essential fats do this job very nicely. As we explored in Chapters 3 and 4, they reduce pain, inflammation and stiffness, inhibit attacks on your joints by the immune system, and provide essential structural materials for the joint membranes. They also help you to stop using pain-killing NSAIDS such as aspirin, which otherwise cause progressive joint damage.

The only problem with essential fats is the large doses required to bring about effective increases in blood levels, a problem that causes some people to skip their essential fats or take amounts insufficient to beat arthritis. At the Colgan Institute, we developed three alternative strategies that suit most folk.

We use **flax oil** to provide basic omega-3 fats. Good flax oil is 50% alpha-linolenic acid, of which about a quarter survives digestion and conversion into the omega-3 fat **eicosapentaenoic acid**, the specific fat that most benefits arthritis.

The effective daily dose of flax oil is 30 – 80 grams (1½ to 4 tablespoons) depending on bodyweight and the patient's arthritis history. A dose of 40 grams (2 tablespoons) is a good average.

Our first strategy, which we advise everyone to follow, is to mix this flax oil in a morning protein shake with fruit and ion-exchange whey protein concentrate. We will see below why that particular protein is best.

An alternative strategy is to blend the flax oil with **quark** (lightly fermented low-fat cottage cheese) and add it to morning cereal. With fruit to taste, it is very palatable, some folk say "delicious." By using quark, which increases omega-3 absorption, you can reduce the dose of flax oil by 25%.

A third strategy is to take your flax oil with balsamic vinegar or other ingredients as a salad dressing or sauce. This mix *is* delicious, especially if you use the right organic flax oil. The best brands are Barleans, Flora, Omega, Arrowhead Mills and Spectrum Naturals.

Some great recipes using flax oil are given in Appendix A. You will see that some of these recipes call for different brands. That's because each brand has its own unique taste, probably depending on the source of the flax. We keep a range of flax oils so we can use the one that suits the recipe best.

To allow for the minority of folk with reduced ability to convert flax oil omega-3s into eicosapentaenoic acid, we add two to eight 1000 milligram capsules per day of **fish oil**, in which the eicosapentaenoic acid comes pre-formed. Four capsules per day, taken as two with your morning shake and two with the evening meal, is effective for most cases.

Getting Your Omega-6's

As we saw in Chapter 3, linoleic acid converts to **gamma-linolenic acid**, the omega-6 fat which most benefits arthritis. The best sources we have found for linoleic acid are **walnut** and **pumpkin seed oils**. The effective dose is 10 – 50 grams, depending on bodyweight and arthritis history. A large tablespoon (20 g) is effective for most folk.

Both walnut and pumpkin seed oils, mixed with different vinegars, make excellent salad dressings. This is the main strategy we advise for using them, because it encourages folk to have a good mixed raw vegetable salad every day. High raw veggie intake is a wise strategy for arthritis because of the wide variety of antioxidant flavonoids and other polyphenols it provides. Other delicious dishes using these oils are given in Appendix A.

To allow for folk whose bodies may have difficulty converting linoleic acid into gamma-linolenic acid, we also use organic **borage oil.** At 24% preformed gamma-linolenic acid, borage oil is the most potent source, much superior to evening primrose (9%) or blackcurrant seed oil (17%). The effective daily dose is four to ten 1000 milligram capsules. Six capsules works for most folk. We advise taking these with your morning shake and with dinner.

For all the oils, you can't go wrong with Barleans, Flora, Omega, Arrowhead Mills or Spectrum Naturals. Some brands such as Flora, Udo's Choice and Omega Essential Balance come ready blended, using the different oils we recommend. Clearly the research supporting their use to promote good health is well known to these manufacturers.

Glucosamine And Chondroitin For Structure

Once you have set the stage for joint repair by changing your diet and supplementing it with essential fats, the next step is to provide your body with preformed **glucosamine**. This substance is the rate-limiting chemical step in the production of **glycosaminoglycans**, the tough, feathery strings that form half the structure of your cartilage. We use only the **glucosamine sulfate** form, because the sulfur it contains is also an essential component for production of glycosaminoglycans.

We also use chondroitin sulfate because of the evidence (reviewed in Chapter 7) that it can help with new collagen formation in cartilage. It may also provide some pre-formed chondroitin-related compounds to cartilage and to synovial fluid.

The effective dose of glucosamine is 2.0 – 8.0 grams per day, depending on bodyweight and arthritis history. Four grams taken in divided doses, morning and evening, is effective for most folk. Best brands are Colgan Institute, Life Extension Foundation, USANA and Twinlabs.

Doses of chondroitin used in research run from 0.5 – 2.0 grams per day. One gram taken in divided doses, morning and evening, is an effective supplement. Best brands are Colgan Institute, Life Extension Foundation and Twinlabs.

SAMe Forms The Keystone

Chapters 8 through 10 relate the great advance in arthritis treatment resulting from our new understanding of **S-adenosylmethionine (SAMe)**. First, SAMe reduces joint inflammation, pain and stiffness, thereby adding to the efficacy of essential fats and further reducing the need for toxic NSAIDS to combat discomfort. Second, SAMe is more efficacious than essential fats in combating auto-immune attacks on your joints, thereby protecting the synovial membrane and your vital synovial fluid (joint oil), so that essential fats can rebuild them.

Third, SAMe protects and restores brain function, thereby relieving the brain poisoning that is the main cause of the depression that plagues folk with many forms of rheumatoid arthritis, osteoarthritis, fibromyalgia and chronic fatigue.

Fourth, SAMe reduces elevated levels of **homocysteine**, now known to damage both brain and joints directly, and also to trigger auto-immune reactions.

The effective daily dose of SAMe is 400 – 1200 milligrams. Partly because of its current high cost, at the Colgan Institute we use a daily minimum of 400 milligrams SAMe, taken in divided doses to enhance absorption.

Folic Acid, Vitamin B₁₂ Vital

As we saw in Chapter 9, folic acid and vitamin B_{12} are essential for conversion of toxic levels of homocysteine back to the non-toxic essential amino acid methionine. Yet in Western Society we are chronically short of these vitamins in our diets. Folk with arthritis should be especially vigilant to get a good supply, as their need is greater than most.

Folic acid and vitamin B_{12} deficiencies both cause brain and joint degeneration, independent of SAMe, homocysteine or anything else. To overcome arthritis and its attendant depression and cognitive problems, eat these vitamins every day.

At the Colgan Institute, we use 0.5 – 10.0 milligrams of folic acid per day depending on bodyweight, arthritis history and blood homocysteine level. A daily dose of 2.0 milligrams is effective for most folk.

We always combine the folic acid with 100 micrograms of vitamin B_{12} per 1.0 milligram of folic acid. This strategy overcomes two problems. First, it ensures that the body has sufficient vitamin B_{12} for the conversion of homocysteine to SAMe. Second, it ensures that folic acid alone does not mask a vitamin B_{12} deficiency, which would then continue to damage both brain and joints.

Antioxidants Beat The Radicals

From Chapter 10 you know that most forms of arthritis involve **uncontrolled oxidation** of the joints. Your joints don't wear out, they "rust" out. This rust can be prevented only by supplementary nutrient **antioxidants**.

Not any old antioxidant will do. You have to neutralize the many different kinds of free radicals step-by-step, by using a wide range of antioxidants to reduce them to harmless carbon dioxide and water. The effective daily mix is given in Chapter 11. The best sources of antioxidants that most closely match this mix are Colgan Institute and Nu-Life-Nu-Sport .

You should divide the daily packet of antioxidants in two, and take half with your morning shake or breakfast and half with the evening meal. Take the melatonin part of the formula at night, within a half hour of bed-time.

Ion-Exchange Whey Protein

We advise all arthritis patients to drink a morning shake made with 10 ounces of non-fat milk, 30 grams **ion-exchange whey protein concentrate**, flax oil, pumpkin oil and fruit to taste. First, the whey concentrate provides extra glutamine for the immune system. In my book, **The New Nutrition,** I show how this food can improve immunity.[1] Second, it provides extra glutamine in just the right form for your body to make glucosamine for the joints. Third, the latest evidence shows that ion-exchange whey has strong antioxidant action.[2] Fourth, as I show in my forthcoming book, **The Sports Nutrition Pocket Guide,** this form of protein has the highest Biological Value for retention of body protein and maintenance of muscle mass.[3] Maintaining muscle is crucial as it is the main source of glutamine that fires your immune system. For all these reasons, ion-exchange whey protein concentrate is a must to beat arthritis.

Buyer beware. In recent tests run by the Colgan Institute, six of eight brands of supposed ion-exchange whey were not true to label. I document elsewhere similar findings by health authorities in Canada and the US.[4] Brands you can trust are Twinlabs Whey Fuel and R_x Fuel, Nu-Life-Nu-Sport Whey More, SISU and Unipro Perfect Protein.

A Typical Day

To help you start on the Road To Happy Joints, Table 3 covers a typical day on the program. With the approval of their physicians, some folk have followed Table 3 religiously for months at a time with spectacular benefits. It is somewhat restrictive, however. There are many delicious foods in Appendix A and numerous alternative ways given in this book to provide your body with the right structural materials. Follow them all and make your life a celebration.

For folk whose work hours, travel schedules, etc, make compliance difficult, the Colgan Institute has developed a Joint Pak which incorporates the major nutrients you need to beat arthritis. Phone 1 (760) 632-7722.

Table 3. Colgan Institute Typical Daily Program to Beat Arthritis

Morning — On Rising

Make a breakfast shake with:

30 g ion-exchange whey protein with soy isoflavones, 10 oz non-fat milk,
2 – 4 tbsp of mixed 50/50 flax and pumpkin seed oil, and fresh fruit to taste.

Take with shake:

- 1 – 2 grams fish oil capsules
- 2 – 3 grams borage oil capsules
- Complete a.m. vitamin/ mineral supplement
- Half of daily antioxidant mix
- Including 200 mg SAMe

- 500 mg chondroitin sulfate
- 2 grams glucosamine sulfate
- 1.0 mg folic acid
- 100 mcg vitamin B_{12}
- 25 mg vitamin B_6
- 25 mg dehydroepiandrosterone (DHEA)

Or Colgan Institute Daily Paks + Joint Pak

Mid-morning — *Gym workout, stretch and water*

Noon

- Scrambled eggs (5 whites with one yolk) on mixed whole-grain toast
- Mixed raw vegetable salad
- Dish of mixed fresh fruit with live low-fat yogurt
- Vegetable juice or herbal tea
- Water

Mid to late afternoon — *Walk 20 – 30 minutes*

Evening

Make dinner with:

Mixed steamed vegetables, 6 – 8 oz of chicken, turkey or ocean fish and whole-grain rolls with a little butter.

Take with dinner:

- 1 – 2 grams fish oil capsules
- 2 – 3 grams borage oil capsules
- Complete p.m. vitamin/ mineral supplement
- Second half of daily antioxidant mix
- Water
- Fruit salad with custard cream

- including 200 mg SAMe
- 2 grams glucosamine sulfate
- 1.0 mg folic acid
- 100 mcg vitamin B_{12}
- 25 mg vitamin B_6
- 500 mg chondroitin sulfate
- Herbal tea
- 1 mg melatonin, within a half hour of bed-time

Or Colgan Institute Daily Paks + Joint Pak

© 1998, The Colgan Institute, San Diego, CA

14

Use It Or Lose It

The final component to the Happy Joints Program is **weight-bearing exercise**. To maintain muscle, bone and the soft tissues between joints, all must be stimulated regularly by moderate weight-bearing stress. Walking, jogging, swimming, tennis or other aerobic exercises are all good fitness activities, but they are not enough to save your joints. Most effective is a regular, moderate weight training regimen. I am pleased to see that exercise programs for arthritis are now turning to weights as the key to long-lasting improvement.[17]

Two recent examples are representative of the evidence in favor of weight training. Dr L C Rall and team at the Human Nutrition Research Center on Aging at Tufts University, compared healthy young people, healthy older people and rheumatoid arthritis patients, who all volunteered for a high-intensity, progressive, resistance exercise program. All three groups demonstrated similar large increases in strength, compared with control subjects who did only light exercise. In addition, all the arthritis patients had significant reductions in pain and fatigue.[1]

Another recent study by Dr J M Schilke and colleagues at the University of Nebraska, examined the effects of an eight-week resistance exercise program on osteoarthritis of the knee. Subjects showed big increases in strength and mobility and big decreases in pain and stiffness. The Osteoarthritis Screening Index showed a large reduction in disease activity.[2]

A pile of recent research confirms these effects. After analyzing more than 100 studies, the Colgan Institute utilized its twenty years of experience in sports training to develop a comprehensive weight training and stretching program that incorporates the best elements of each. We have used it with great success. The basic principles are detailed below. You should take this program to your physician and get their approval to use it too.

Please, please develop the habit of regular resistance exercise. If you don't, two big chunks of evidence fairly shout that you will never attain happy joints. First, the medical literature shows that folk with arthritis do less exercise than average.[8] And folk with arthritis are weaker than average,[9,10] despite the clear evidence that muscle strength alleviates this group of diseases.[1-7]

Second, important new research shows that unless you stimulate your body to heal, nutritional supplement programs have little effect. A representative study published in the New England Journal of Medicine, showed that a multi-vitamin/mineral program yielded only minor improvements in the health of older folk. But when a weight-bearing exercise program was added, health and well being, strength and mobility improved dramatically.[11]

The principles of weight training are covered in detail in my books, **The New Nutrition** and **Optimum Sports Nutrition**.[12,13] The exact ways to do weight exercises are covered in my forthcoming book **The Power Program**.[14] The principles you need to know when exercising specifically to beat arthritis are:

1. **Professional Help**

   First, obtain a clearance to do this program of weight exercise from your physician. Then enroll at a gym and take some sessions with a certified trainer who will show you the correct form for the following exercises. Correct form is essential when lifting weights in order to protect your joints. Do *not* try to learn on your own.

2. **Not Aerobics**

   Do *not* take the usual aerobic classes in the vain hope of losing weight, maintaining muscle or helping your joints. The Colgan Institute and other researchers have shown repeatedly that they do not work.[12] Yet, despite the evidence, every day at almost every gym I know, you are greeted by an ocean of beefy booties, all bobbing furiously to the latest beat. They seem to have the mistaken idea that if they jiggle their fat up and down long enough it will somehow fall off.

3. **Not Bodybuilding**

   Do *not* follow the weight regimens of bodybuilders. Many of these folk so overstress their joints they are continually consulting the Colgan Institute for help with joint and connective tissue injuries. In later life, arthritis will visit them savagely. You will recognize them in the gym. Do not exercise like anyone you see grunting under heavy piles of iron, who is so overbuilt he resembles an agitated haggis with a varicose problem.

4. **Specific Exercises Only**
    Do only the exercises listed here. Many common weight exercises are dangerous for anyone with compromised joints. Never do barbell pulls up to the chin for example, or lying dumbbell pullovers, or barbell squats, as they are murder on the shoulders, neck, knees and lower back of anyone with arthritis.

5. **Always Warm Up**
    Warm up all your muscles and joints thoroughly for 15 minutes using a cross-country machine or a rowing machine. The rule is: *Never touch a weight 'til you break a sweat.* Do *not* use a stationery bike, *nor* a treadmill *nor* a stair stepper or stair climber, as these warm up only a restricted number of muscles and joints.

6. **Drink Water**
    Keep a water bottle with you throughout gym workouts and sip frequently. You should consume at least one liter of water per workout.

7. **Three Workouts A Week**
    Do weight training **three** days per week, preferably Monday, Wednesday and Friday.

8. **Specific Bodyparts**
    Mondays: do shoulders and arms. Wednesdays: do chest and back. Fridays: do legs and abdominals.

9. **Supersets**
    For arthritis it is best to do exercises in pairs called **supersets**. That is, you do a set of the first exercise followed by a set of the second. Ideally, the second exercise of each pair contracts opposing muscles to those contracted by the first exercise and moves the joints in the opposite direction.

Example: A set of standing dumbbell curls, which exercise the biceps and bend the arm at the elbow, should be followed immediately by a set of dumbbell kickbacks which exercise the triceps and straighten the arm at the elbow.

10. Two Sets

Do **two** sets per exercise.

Set 1. Use a light to medium weight for **12 – 15** repetitions.

Set 2. Use a medium to moderately heavy weight for **6 – 10** repetitions.

11. Acceleration Then Deceleration

Accelerate the concentric contraction and decelerate the eccentric contraction of each repetition. That is, lift the weight quickly (while remaining in good form) when the muscle is shortening under the load. Then lower the weight slowly when the muscle is lengthening under the load.

Example: In a bicep curl, curl the barbell quickly to the chest, then lower it slowly. The relative counts should be one elephant, two elephants up, one elephant, two elephants, three elephants, four elephants down.

12. Full Range of Motion

Always use the full range of motion of the joint with each exercise.

13. Breathe

Do *not* hold your breath while lifting a weight, a common and dangerous fault. Take a deep breath in and exhale slowly while lifting until fully exhaled at the top of the lift. Then take another deep breath in and exhale slowly while lowering the weight.

14. Length of Workout

Workouts vary in length: 10 exercises in Workout 1, six in Workout 2, and eight in Workout 3, depending on muscle size and type. The longest workout should not take you more than 45 minutes. The Exercise Program is pictured and described overleaf.

15. Stretch

Stretch for 10 minutes immediately after your weight workout. The Stretch Program is pictured and described directly after the Exercise Program.

16. Get a copy of the **Colgan Institute Power Program.** This companion book allows you to record your weight training on charts containing all the above exercises. It comes complete with a full description and photographic guide to each exercise, plus many more exercises and a full stretching program. For those who want the ultimate guide, you can also get the **Colgan Institute Power Program Video,** in which my team and I demonstrate the precise form of each exercise and stretch. Both are available from Apple Publishing at 1-800-668-2775.

17. Above all, start easy. Use only the weights you can handle with comfort. Contrary to all those machismo advertisements for fitness, your body does *not* have to become inflamed in order to improve. *Start ea-s-s-s-y!*

Workout 1: Shoulders and Arms

Shoulders: Alternate each set of Exercise 1 with a set of Exercise 2.

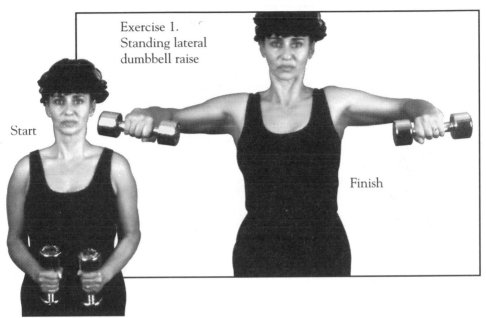

Exercise 1.
Standing lateral
dumbbell raise

Start

Finish

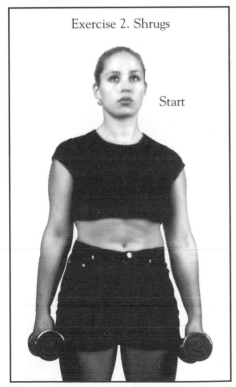
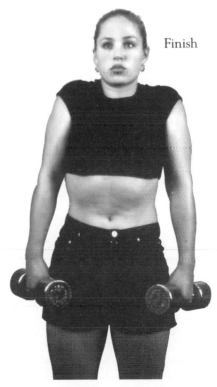

Exercise 2. Shrugs

Start

Finish

Workout 1: Shoulders and Arms (cont'd)

Shoulders: Alternate each set of Exercise 3 with a set of Exercise 4.

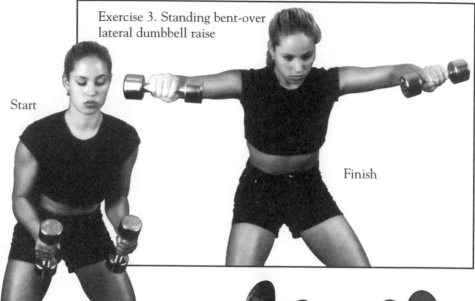

Exercise 3. Standing bent-over lateral dumbbell raise

Start

Finish

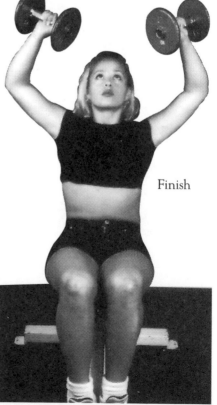

Exercse 4. Seated dumbbell press above head with elbows back

Start

Finish

Workout 1: Shoulders and Arms (con'd)

Arms: Alternate each set of Exercise 5 with a set of Exercise 6.

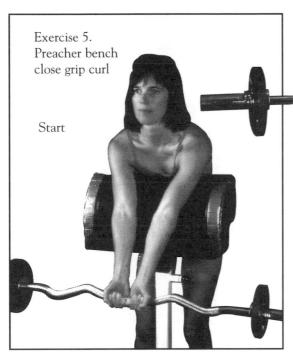

Exercise 5.
Preacher bench
close grip curl

Start

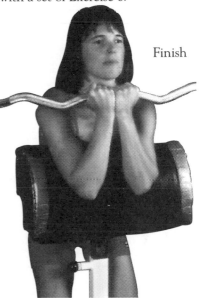

Finish

Exercise 6. Triceps pushdown
with V-bar

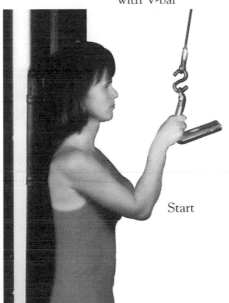

Start

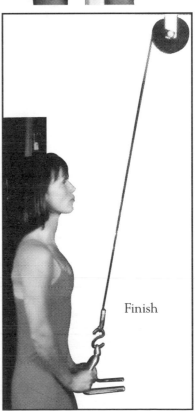

Finish

Workout 1: Shoulders and Arms (con'd)

Arms: Alternate each set of Exercise 7 with a set of Exercise 8.

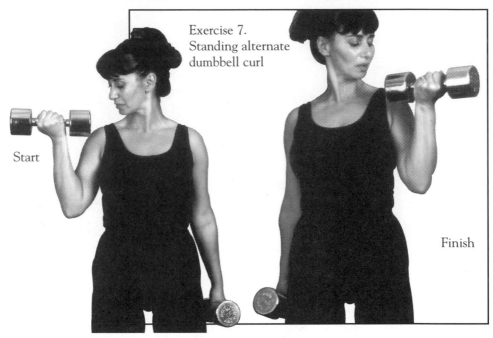

Exercise 7.
Standing alternate
dumbbell curl

Start

Finish

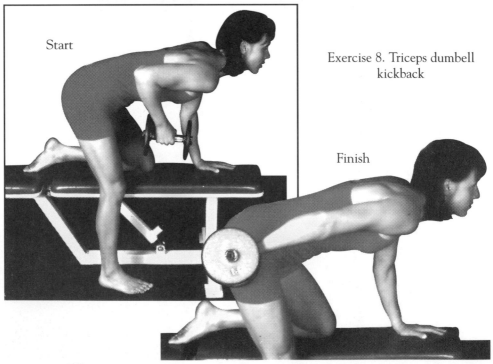

Start

Exercise 8. Triceps dumbell
kickback

Finish

Workout 1: Shoulders and Arms (cont'd)

Arms: Alternate each set of Exercise 9 with a set of Exercise 10.

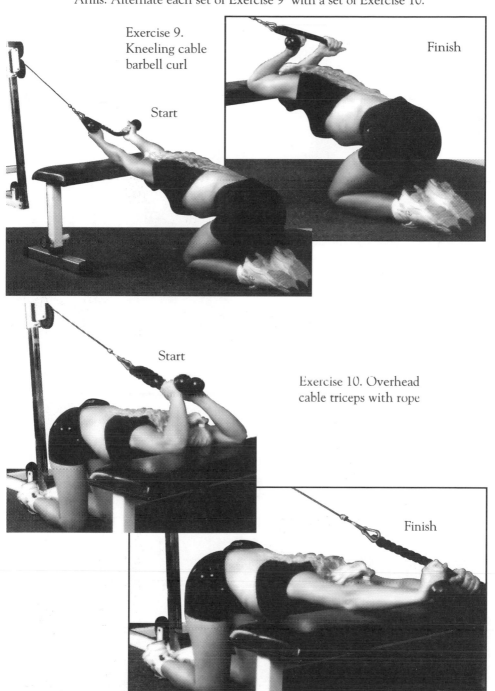

Exercise 9.
Kneeling cable
barbell curl

Finish

Start

Start

Exercise 10. Overhead
cable triceps with rope

Finish

Workout 2: Chest and Back

Chest and Back: Alternate each set of Exercise 1 with a set of Exercise 2

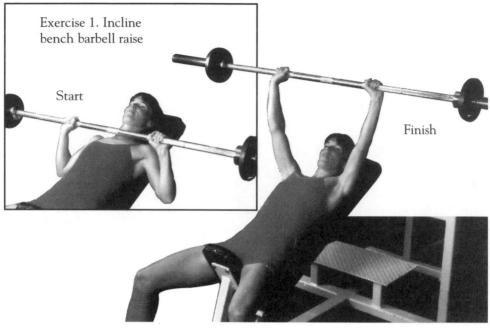

Exercise 1. Incline
bench barbell raise

Start

Finish

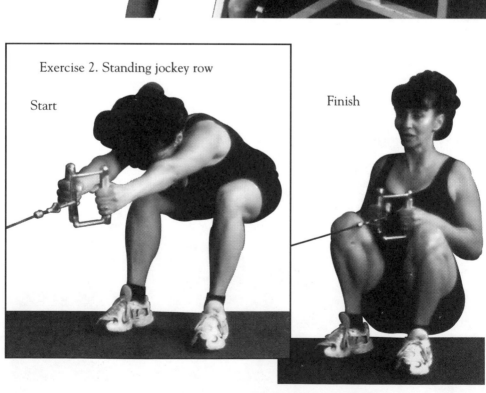

Exercise 2. Standing jockey row

Start

Finish

Workout 2: Chest and Back (cont'd)

Chest and Back: Alternate each set of Exercise 3 with a set of Exercise 4.

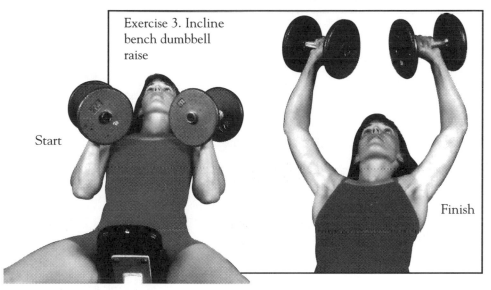

Exercise 3. Incline bench dumbbell raise

Start

Finish

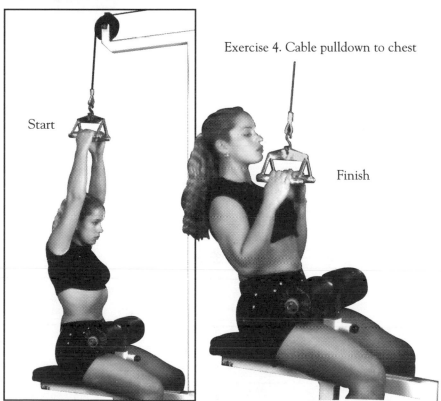

Start

Exercise 4. Cable pulldown to chest

Finish

Workout 2: Chest and Back (cont'd)

Chest and Back: Alternate each set of Exercise 5 with a set of Exercise 6.

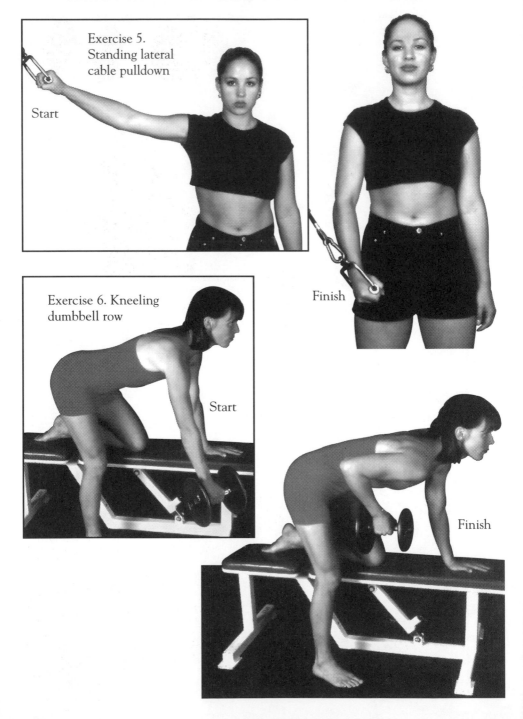

Exercise 5.
Standing lateral
cable pulldown

Start

Finish

Exercise 6. Kneeling
dumbbell row

Start

Finish

Workout 3: Legs, Abdominals, Lower Back

Legs: Alternate each set of Exercise 1 with a set of Exercise 2.

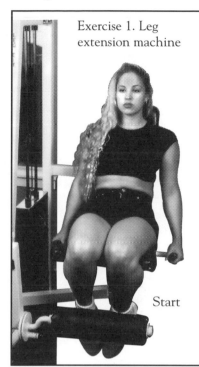
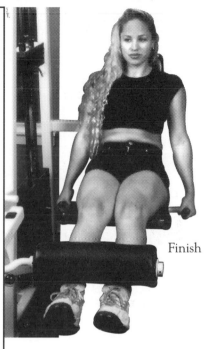

Exercise 1. Leg extension machine

Start

Finish

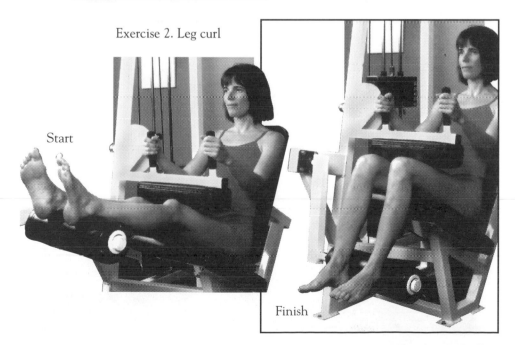

Exercise 2. Leg curl

Start

Finish

Workout 3: Legs, Abdominals, Lower Back (cont'd)

Legs: Alternate each set of Exercise 3 with a set of Exercise 4.

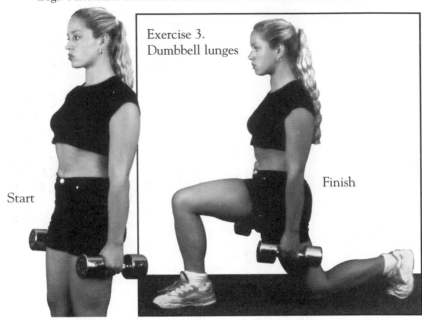

Exercise 3.
Dumbbell lunges

Start

Finish

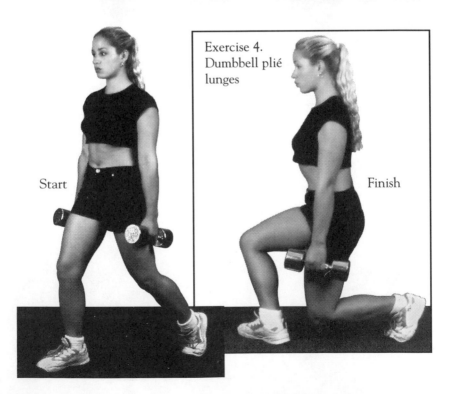

Exercise 4.
Dumbbell plié
lunges

Start

Finish

Workout 3: Legs, Abdominals, Lower Back (cont'd)

Abs and Back: Alternate each set of Exercise 5 with a set of Exercise 6.

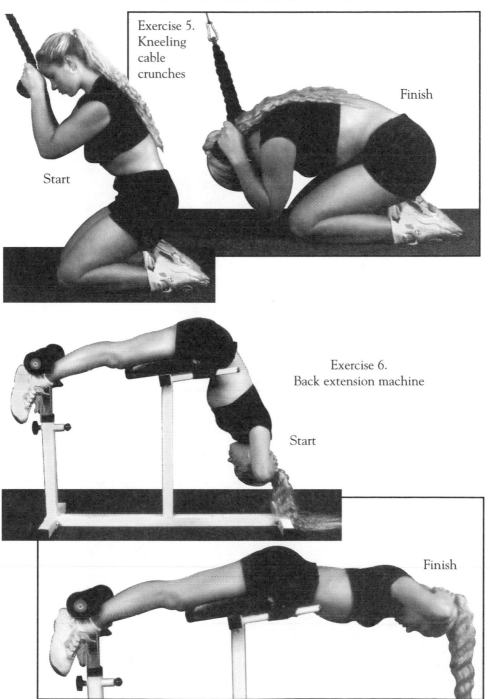

Exercise 5.
Kneeling
cable
crunches

Finish

Start

Exercise 6.
Back extension machine

Start

Finish

Workout 3: Legs, Abdominals, Lower Back (cont'd)

Abs and Back: Alternate each set of Exercise 7 with a set of Exercise 8.

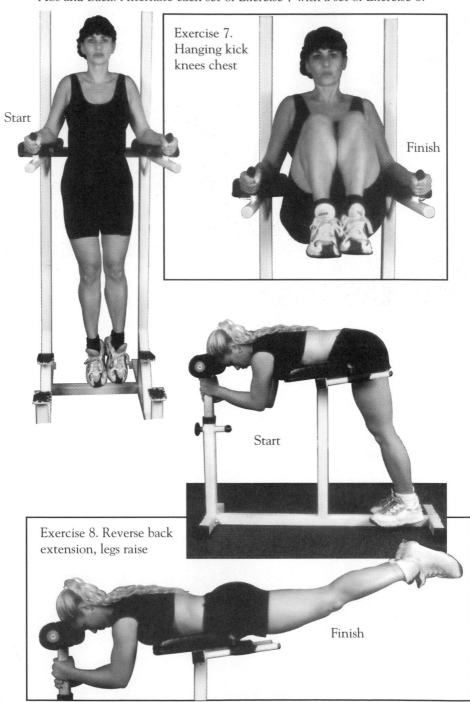

Exercise 7.
Hanging kick
knees chest

Start

Finish

Start

Exercise 8. Reverse back
extension, legs raise

Finish

Effective Stretching

1. **Never stretch cold.** Stretch gently after your workout, while your body is still warm and sweating. Stretching in a hot tub or in a shower with hot water playing on the stretch is the optimum.

2. **Never bounce.** Bouncing into a stretch, though popular in some gyms, results in shorter, tighter muscles, tendons and ligaments, that set you up for injury.

3. **Never force.** The groans heard from people stretching in gyms are a sure signal of disaster. Stretch only to the point of pressure, never to the point of pain. Pushing to pain brings only inflammation and injury. You will not be able to copy the photographs right away. Be patient. In six months, your progress will amaze you.

4. **Relax.** Especially keep your face, jaw and shoulders relaxed, as these areas are the first to tense during effort. Concentrate on relaxing the stretching muscles. Ease slowly into the stretch. If the muscles tighten and pull against the stretch, ease out of it until they relax. Otherwise you are creating shorter, tighter muscles and inviting connective tissue injury. This is the most common fault which prevents folk becoming flexible by stretching, and which persuades some that stretching exercises are ineffective.

5. **Breathe.** Take deep, slow, even breaths throughout stretching. Breathe out as you move smoothly into the maximum stretch position. Back off a little and breathe in. Then breathe out as you move smoothly back into the maximum stretch position.

6. **Articulate.** At the point of stretch, rotate the limbs in and out, especially at hips and shoulders. This articulation of the joint at maximum extension is a big secret of success in stretching to beat arthritis.

7. **Hold each stretch** for 30 – 60 seconds, about four to eight slow breaths. Move into the stretch four times as you exhale, and back off each time you inhale.

8. **Patience.** Good flexibility takes years to accomplish. Every time you force a stretch, you inhibit progress. The six keys to success are: warmth, smooth movement, relaxation, breathing, articulation and patience. You can do it.

Stretches For Happy Joints

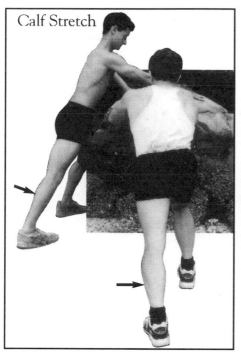

Calf Stretch

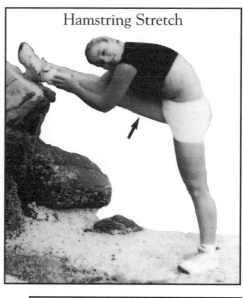

Hamstring Stretch

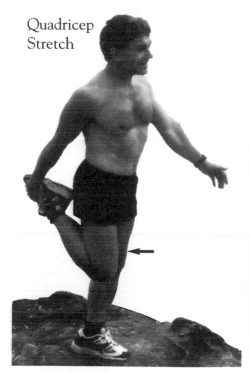

Quadricep Stretch

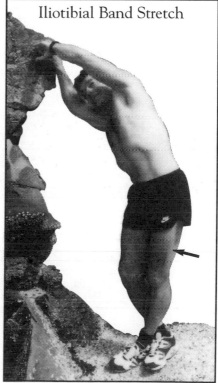

Iliotibial Band Stretch

Stretches for Happy Joints (cont'd)

Hip Stretch No. 1

Shoulder Stretch

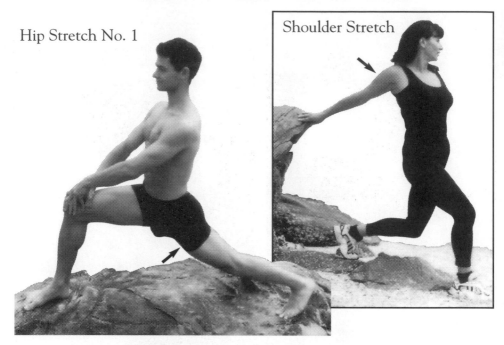

Back Stretch

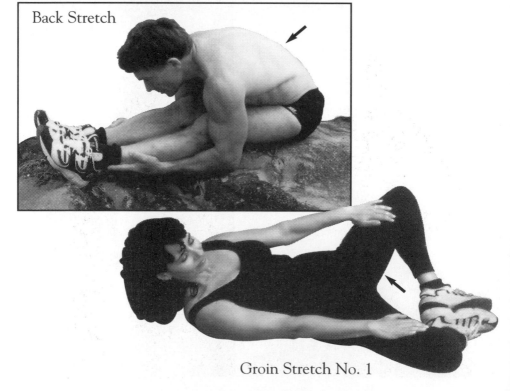

Groin Stretch No. 1

Stretches for Happy Joints (cont'd)

Hip Stretch No. 2

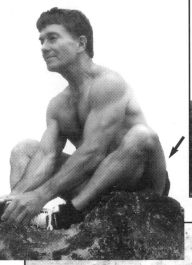

Hip Stretch No. 3

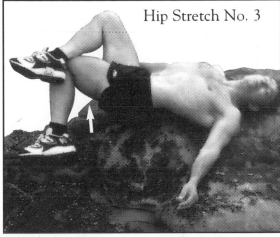

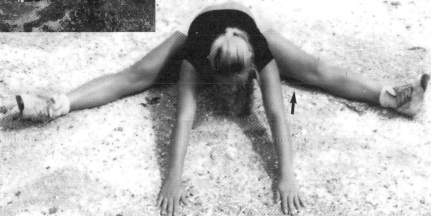

Back Stretch

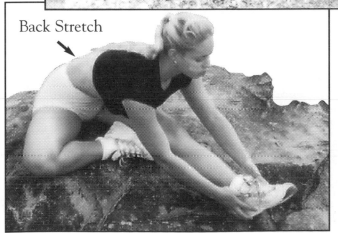

Groin Stretch No. 2

Stretches for Happy Joints (cont'd)

Lower Back
Stretch No. 1

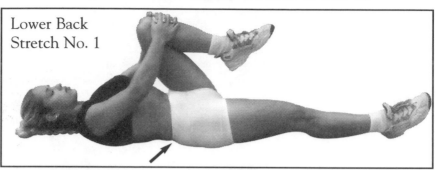

Hip and Back Stretch

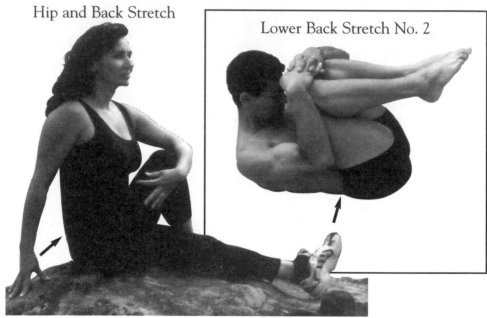

Lower Back Stretch No. 2

Groin Stretch No. 3

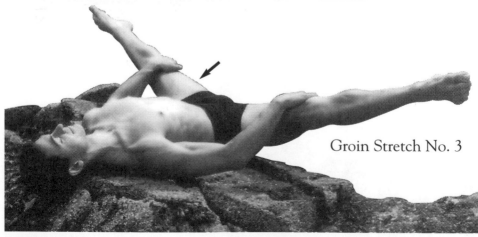

At 60 years of age, Dr. Michael Colgan is living proof of the effectiveness of his nutritional and exercise programs for maintaining muscle and flexibility, and preventing disease and degeneration.

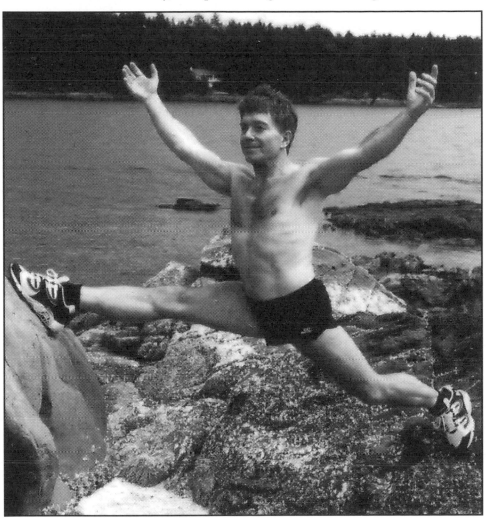

Swansong

All that remains is to wish you Godspeed on your journey to beat arthritis. You should also use the wonderful recipes given in Appendix A. They are not mine, but have been donated by patients, friends and gourmet chefs. Enjoy them in the certain knowledge that they are helping to guide your way to health and vitality.

Freedom from pain and illness is the finest state of being. It enables you to concentrate your time and attention on what is most important in life. Come join me in the 21st century in joy and fulfillment.

> Practice excellence in everything you do,
> And excellence will grow within your mind.
>
> Practice closeness towards all those that you love,
> And love will flourish in your heart.
>
> Practice compassion towards everyone you meet,
> And nobility will come to fill your spirit.
>
> Then the purpose of life is bound to your being,
> And its realization shines from your eyes.
>
> Michael Colgan,
> July, 1998.

Appendix A
Gourmet Foods For Joints

Eating is one of life's great pleasures. Yet so-called "healthy" eating is often viewed as insipid and unsatisfying. I have spent three decades in pursuit of those folk who realize that God dwells in the details, and have applied that realization to refine healthy meals so that they become gourmet treats. Here are some of my finds.

These meals are not meant to be a complete list. They are just some tempting samples of the quickest, easiest and most delicious recipes that friends and patients, including great chefs, have given to us in appreciation. These particular foods fit well into the Beat Arthritis Program. Enjoy them, as we do. May the succulent juices of culinary satisfaction forever run down your chin.

Essential Muesli
*Essential fats, whole grains
and nutrients that increase their absorption.*

Serves Four

Ingredients

4 tbsp	Pumpkin seeds
4 tbsp	Sesame seeds
4 tbsp	Sunflower seeds
4 tbsp	Flaxseed
2 tbsp	Almonds with skins
4 cups	Rolled oats
½ cup	Fresh apple juice
to taste	Cinnamon
1 cup	Fresh fruit
1 cup	Plain low-fat quark

Instructions

- Grind pumpkin seeds, sesame seeds, sunflower seeds and flaxseed lightly in a coffee grinder.
- Chop almonds.
- Combine nuts and seeds with oats.
- Stir in apple juice.
- Add cinnamon and fresh fruit.
- Let stand five minutes.
- Top with quark and serve.

Lifeshake
Consider this shake your daily body armour against arthritis.

Serves One

Ingredients

10 oz	Non-fat milk
30 g	Ion-exchange whey protein concentrate with soy isoflavones
1 tbsp	Barleans's flax oil
1 tbsp	Organic pumpkin seed oil
1 cup	Fresh fruit, chopped

Instructions

- Blend ingredients at high speed.
- Drink immediately.

Instead of the flax oil and pumpkin seed oil you can use 2 tbsp of Omega Essential Balance *or* 2 tbsp of Flora Udo's Choice.

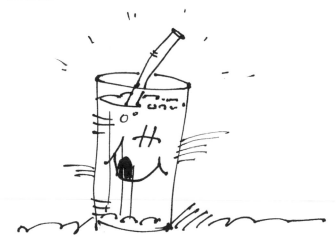

Humpty's Hummus
A healthier variation on the traditional Middle Eastern dish used as a dip or as a filling in pita sandwiches.

Makes about Three Cups

Ingredients

2 cups	Canned organic garbanzo beans
¼ cup	Tahini (sesame seed paste)
3 tbsp	Lemon juice
2 tbsp	Organic flax oil
1 tbsp	Organic pumpkin seed oil
2	Organic garlic cloves
¼ tsp	Ground coriander
¼ tsp	Ground cumin
¼ tsp	Paprika
dash	Cayenne
1 tbsp	Minced scallions
2 tbsp	Minced fresh parsley

Instructions

- Blend garbanzo beans, tahini, lemon juice, flax oil and pumpkin seed oil until the mixture reaches the consistency of a coarse paste. Use garbanzo liquid from can only as needed.
- Add garlic, coriander, cumin, paprika and cayenne. Blend thoroughly.
- Transfer hummus to a bowl and stir in scallions.
- Cover and refrigerate.
- Garnish with parsley when serving.

Instead of the flax and pumpkin oils, you can use 3 tbsp of Omega Essential Balance or 3 tbsp of Flora Udo's Choice.

Domino's Angel Hair
Pasta that tastes like nutty silk.

Serves Four

Ingredients

8 oz	Organic angel hair pasta
3 large	Italian tomatoes, chopped into ½ inch cubes
1 large	Organic garlic clove, crushed
1 cup	Chopped fresh basil
¼ tsp	Potassium/sodium ½ and ½ salt
to taste	Freshly ground black pepper
2 tbsp	Barlean's flax oil

Instructions

- Prepare pasta according to package directions.
- While pasta cooks, prepare sauce.
- Combine the tomatoes, garlic, basil, salt and pepper. Add the flax oil and whisk well.
- Add half the sauce to hot pasta and mix.
- Top with the remaining sauce and serve.

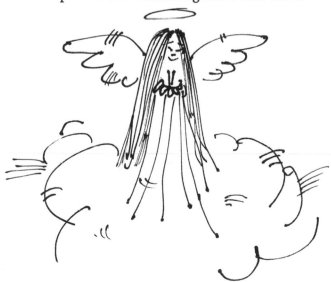

Mi Piace Spaghetti Marinara
Serves Four

Ingredients

1 lb	Organic semolina spaghetti
1 tbsp	Extra virgin olive oil
¾ cup	Chopped white onion
⅓ cup	Chopped celery
⅓ cup	Chopped carrot
1 large	Clove garlic, crushed
1 tbsp	Nutritional yeast
6 large	Italian tomatoes, peeled and chopped
¼ tsp	Dried oregano
¼ tsp	Dried basil
pinch	Potassium/sodium ½ and ½ salt
to taste	Freshly ground black pepper
1 tbsp	Tomato paste
1 tbsp	Arrowhead Mills flax oil

Instructions

- Prepare spaghetti according to package directions.
- While spaghetti cooks, prepare sauce.
- Heat olive oil in a medium pan. Add onion, celery, carrot and garlic. Sauté over medium heat for three minutes, stirring frequently.
- Add the yeast and stir well.
- Add tomatoes, oregano, basil, salt and pepper. Stir in tomato paste. Cover and simmer over low heat, stirring occasionally until sauce becomes uniform in consistency, about 20 minutes.
- Remove from heat and stir in flax oil.
- Add half sauce to spaghetti and stir in.
- Top with remaining sauce and serve.

Barleans or Flora flax oil will also work well in this recipe.

Lip-smacking Lemon Chicken

Serves Four

Ingredients

½ cup	Fresh squeezed lemon juice
1	Clove garlic, chopped
pinch	Pepper
4	Fresh boneless chicken breasts
3 sprigs	Fresh rosemary
1	Lemon, thinly sliced

Instructions

- Combine lemon juice, garlic and pepper.
- Place chicken in one layer on bottom of shallow dish.
- Pour juice mixture over chicken and turn to thoroughly coat both sides.
- Pull rosemary needles off sprigs and sprinkle over chicken.
- Let stand for 15 minutes.
- Grill chicken over high heat for about five minutes per side, until meat at center is no longer pink.
- Garnish with lemon slices and serve.

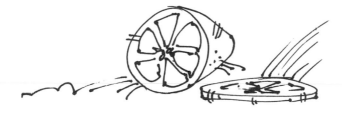

Chicken Jig-Jig
Like South Sea Islands sunshine.

Serves Four

Ingredients

3 tbsp	Brown sugar
½ tsp	Nutmeg
¼ tsp	Cinnamon
¼ tsp	Pepper
¼ tsp	Allspice
¼ cup	Fresh squeezed lime juice
6	Boneless, skinless chicken breasts
1 tbsp	Omega Essential Balance Oil
2 tbsp	Water or chicken broth
2 tbsp	Sherry
2 tbsp	White wine
¼ cup	Marjoram, chopped
2 tbsp	Sage, chopped
½ cup	Pineapple, chopped

Instructions

- Combine first six ingredients.
- Brown chicken in skillet over high heat.
- Reduce heat, brush both sides of chicken with oil and cook another 10 minutes.
- Put chicken aside and keep warm.
- Add broth to herb/sugar mixture, cook two minutes.
- Add remaining ingredients, reduce heat.
- Add chicken and baste with sauce.
- Cover and simmer on low heat for 10 minutes.
- Serve with mixed brown and wild rice.

Ollie's Turkey Tempter

High in protein, low in fat, quick to make and scrumptious.

Serves Four

Ingredients

2 tbsp	Grated orange peel
1 cup	Fresh squeezed orange juice
1	Clove garlic, crushed
1 tbsp	Fresh tarragon
1 lb	Fresh turkey breast, thinly sliced
1	Peeled orange, thinly sliced

Instructions

- Combine orange juice, orange peel, garlic and tarragon.
- Place sequential layers of turkey slice on bottom of shallow dish. Cover each layer with juice mixture.
- Let stand 10 minutes.
- Grill over high heat for two minutes per side.
- Garnish with orange slices and serve.

Halibut In Heaven
You can also use sea bass or cod.

Serves Four

Ingredients

2 cups	Organic tomatoes, finely diced
½ cup	Organic cucumber, finely diced
½ cup	Organic red onion, finely diced
¼ cup	Organic dill, finely chopped
1 tbsp	Barlean's flax oil
1 tbsp	Organic pumpkin seed oil
½ cup	Rice vinegar
½ cup	Fresh squeezed lemon juice
to taste	White pepper
1 lb	Fresh halibut fillet

Instructions

- Combine all ingredients except halibut and let stand 30 – 60 minutes in refrigerator.
- Grill halibut until flesh turns opaque and flakes, 10 – 20 minutes depending on thickness of fillet.
- Pour vegetable mixture over fish and serve.

Alternative brands of flax oil that work well in this recipe are Flora and Omega.

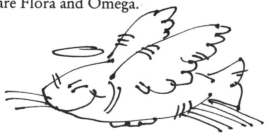

Salmon Delight

Brings back wild days of salmon fishing in the Queen Charlotte Islands off Western Canada.

Serves Four

Ingredients

1 cup	Fresh shallots, minced
2 cups	Field mushrooms, thinly sliced
2 tbsp	Extra virgin olive oil
¼ cup	Fresh dill, chopped
¼ cup	Fresh squeezed lemon juice
to taste	Fresh ground pepper
pinch	Potassium/sodium ½ and ½ salt
1 large	Papaya, sliced
1 tbsp	White wine vinegar
1 lb	Fillet of fresh coho or chinook salmon
1	Lemon, thinly sliced

Instructions

- Combine shallots and mushrooms, olive oil, dill, lemon juice, salt and pepper to taste. Let stand 5 minutes.
- Combine papaya slices with vinegar, salt and pepper to taste. Let stand.
- Lightly oil fish with olive oil and place in shallow dish, skin down.
- Pour shallot/mushroom mixture thickly over fish. Arrange lemon slices along length.
- Bake in oven for 20 minutes at 400° F (200°).
- Transfer to serving dish, garnish with papaya mixture and serve.

Pancho Villa Salsa

*Great as a dip for tortilla chips or as a sauce on enchiladas,
burritos and tacos. Olé!*

Makes Two Cups

Ingredients

3	Tomatoes, diced
4 sprigs	Fresh cilantro
½ med	Onion, diced
1	Scallion, chopped
1 small	Jalapeño pepper
½ cup	Tomato sauce
1 tbsp	Barlean's flax oil
1 tbsp	Organic pumpkin seed oil

Instructions

- Combine tomatoes, cilantro, onion, scallion and jalapeño pepper in a blender and blend to desired consistency, chunky or smooth.
- In a separate bowl, combine tomato sauce, flax oil and pumpkin seed oil. Stir to a uniform consistency.
- Mix everything together and chill until ready to serve.

Instead of flax oil and pumpkin seed oil, you can use 2 tbsp of Omega Essential Balance or 2 tbsp of Udo's Choice.

Awesome Onion Sauce

A treat over steamed veggies or artichokes, and as a dip for the raw veggie plate.

Makes 1 ½ Cups

Ingredients

2 tbsp	Extra virgin olive oil
1 large	White onion, diced
¼ tsp	Ground thyme
1 cup	Water
3 tsp	Organic miso
2 tbsp	Flora flax oil

Instructions

- Heat olive oil in a skillet. Add onion and thyme. Sauté, stirring for three to four minutes, until onion begins to brown.
- Add water and miso. Bring to a boil and simmer three to four minutes over high heat.
- Purée in a blender. Add flax oil and blend to combine.
- Use immediately or refrigerate for later use that day. Can be heated gently.

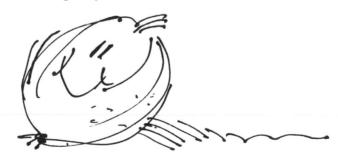

Mama's M'mm Mushroom Gravy
For everywhere that gravy goes.

Makes 2½ Cups

Ingredients

1 tbsp	Extra virgin olive oil
1	White onion, diced
1	Clove of garlic, crushed
1½ cups	Sliced mushrooms
1 tbsp	Whole wheat flour
¼ tsp	Ground thyme
1 tsp	Nutritional yeast
1½ cups	Water
1½ tbsp	Organic vegetable broth powder
2½ tbsp	Arrowhead Mills flax oil

Instructions

- Heat olive oil in a pot. Add onion and garlic and sauté until soft, about three to four minutes.
- Add mushrooms and sauté two to three minutes, stirring occasionally.
- Stir in flour, thyme and yeast. Slowly add water, stirring with a whisk until smooth.
- Add vegetable broth powder and continue to stir. Allow gravy to simmer and thicken over medium heat for about five minutes.
- Remove from heat and cool to serving temperature.
- Stir in flax oil and serve.

Val's Vitality Dressing
A rich, creamy and tasty alternative to commercial mayonnaise.

Makes One Cup

Ingredients

¼ cup	Organic raw almonds
¼ cup	Soy milk or rice milk
½ tsp	Nutritional yeast
¼ tsp	Garlic powder
¼ cup	Omega flax oil
¼ cup	Organic pumpkin seed oil
¼ cup	Extra virgin olive oil
2 tbsp	Lemon juice
¼ tsp	Balsamic vinegar

Instructions

- Starting with almonds, combine ingredients one by one in a blender in the order given above.
- Refrigerate until ready to use. Keeps for 10 days refrigerated.

Sunshine Seed Dressing
Get your essential oils the gourmet way.

Makes about Two Cups

Ingredients

½ cup	Flora Udo's Choice oil
1 cup	Hulled sunflower seeds
¼ cup	Lemon juice
½ cup	Soft tofu
1 tbsp	Low-salt soy sauce
½ tsp	Dried basil
½ tsp	Dried thyme
½ tbsp	Water, as required

Instructions

- Combine all ingredients in a blender or food processor and blend until creamy.
- Refrigerate. Keeps three days.

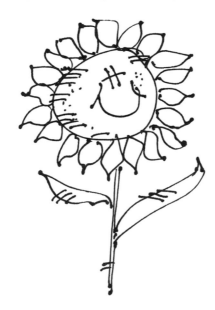

Tangy-Tarragon Dressing

Makes ½ Cup

Ingredients

¼ cup	Fresh squeezed lemon juice
2 tbsp	Water
1 tsp	Dijon mustard
pinch	Cayenne
2 tbsp	Barlean's flax oil
1 tbsp	Fresh tarragon

Instructions

- Combine lemon juice, water, mustard and cayenne in a blender and blend.
- Add flax oil and tarragon and blend well.
- Refrigerate. Keeps 10 days.

Gargantuan Garlic Dressing

A dairyless salad dressing that mimics the richness and texture of sour cream. Great on baked yams and potatoes.

Makes 1 ½ Cups

Ingredients

2 tbsp	Barlean's flax oil
1 tbsp	Organic pumpkin seed oil
¼ cup	Water
2 tbsp	White miso
1 tbsp	Tahini
2 large	Cloves garlic, chopped
1 tbsp	Fresh ginger, peeled and chopped
1 tbsp	Lemon juice

Instructions

- Combine all ingredients in a blender and blend until creamy.
- Cover and refrigerate for use in next 3 days.

Instead of the flax oil and pumpkin seed oil you can use 3 tbsp of Omega Essential Balance or 3 tbsp of Udo's Choice.

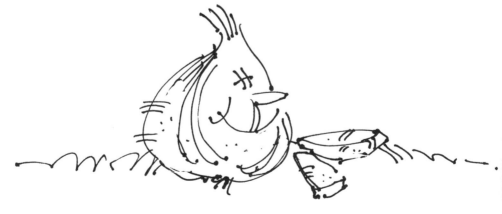

Olympus Dressing
On fresh, organic vegetable salad, a taste of Greek Gods.

Makes One Cup

Ingredients

½ cup	Omega Essential Balance Oil
¼ cup	Red wine vinegar
¼ cup	Feta cheese, finely crumbled
1 or 2	Cloves garlic, minced
1 tbsp	Dijon-style mustard
2 tbsp	Fresh thyme, chopped
1 tbsp	Fresh marjoram, chopped
1 tbsp	Fresh oregano, chopped
1 tsp	Organic honey
¼ tsp	Pepper
to taste	Salt

Instructions

- Place all ingredients in jar, seal tightly.
- Shake vigorously until mixed.
- Use immediately or refrigerate.
- Will keep up to two weeks refrigerated.

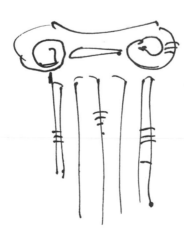

Peter's Perfect Peachy Pie
Just peachy!

Makes One Pie

Ingredients

1	Organic wholewheat piecrust
5 to 6	Large peaches, peeled
3 tbsp	Fresh orange juice
½ cup	Raw whole cashew nuts
3 tbsp	Organic maple syrup
½ cup	Water
1 tsp	Vanilla extract
½ cup	Flora flax oil
1 cup	Low fat quark or yoghurt

Instructions

- Bake piecrust to golden brown.
- Slice peaches thinly.
- Mix peaches with orange juice and set aside.
- Blend cashews in a blender with maple syrup, water and vanilla, until creamy and smooth.
- With blender running on low speed, add flax oil in a thin stream until the mixture thickens.
- Coat bottom of piecrust with a thin layer of cashew mixture. Add a layer of peach slices in a flower petal fashion. Spread with cashew mixture and continue layering, ending with a top layer of peaches.
- Refrigerate for at least two hours.
- Top with quark or yoghurt, and serve.

Raspberry Cream Delight
Lipsmacking!

Serves Four to Six

Ingredients

3 cups	Fresh organic raspberries
2 cups	Low-fat vanilla quark or yoghurt
½ cup	Ion-exchange whey protein concentrate
1 tbsp	Fresh-squeezed lemon juice
1 tbsp	Barlean's flax oil

Instructions

- Purée raspberries in blender, then sieve to remove seeds.
- Blend quark, protein concentrate, lemon juice and flax oil until smooth.
- Add raspberry purée.
- Put in ice cream maker and freeze.
- Serve.

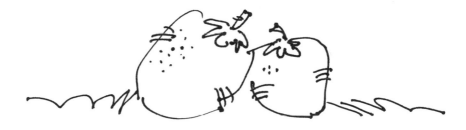

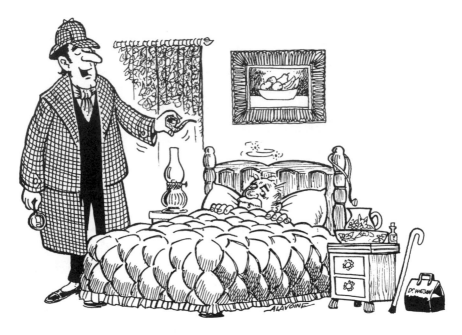

"Alimentary my dear Watson!"

Appendix B
About
Dr. Colgan

Michael Colgan, PhD, CCN, is a renowned lecturer and author of numerous books and articles on nutrition, sports performance and inhibition of aging.

From 1971 to 1982, he was a senior member of the Science Faculty at the University of Auckland, New Zealand. There, he taught in both Human Sciences and the Medical School, while conducting research on human aging and physical performance.

From 1980 to 1982, Dr Colgan was a visiting scholar at Rockefeller University in New York. He has also lectured at Oxford University in England, the University of California in San Diego and the University of Oregon in Washington.

Dr Colgan's professional memberships include the American College of Sports Medicine, the New York Academy of Sciences, the British Society for Nutritional Medicine and the American Academy of Anti-Aging Medicine. He is on the Council of International and American Association of Clinical Nutritionists (the US certification authority for clinical nutritionists), and the Editorial Board of the Journal of Applied Nutrition.

Since 1979, Dr Colgan has been Director of the Colgan Institute.

THE COLGAN INSTITUTE

The Colgan Institute was formed in Auckland, New Zealand, in 1974. In 1982, its head office and laboratory were relocated to San Diego, California.

The Colgan Institute is a consulting, education and research facility, concerned with the effects of nutrition and exercise on sports performance and inhibition of aging.

The Institute has published numerous professional papers, two university texts, five books and over 300 popular articles. It also publishes a monthly magazine, **The Colgan Chronicles**, which has subscribers throughout the world.

In the areas of sports nutrition and longevity, the Institute provides services to major manufacturers and to government in:

- human nutrition research;
- reviews of advances in nutrition;
- analysis of market trends in nutrition; and,
- design of nutritional formulations.

The Institute's clients include, the US National Institute on Aging, the New Zealand Government, and numerous companies including Twinlabs, Weider Health & Fitness, Gull Laboratories, USANA, Nu-Life, Dupont and Digital Equipment.

For the public, the Colgan Institute provides:

- individual nutrition and exercise programs;
- nutrition education programs; and,
- nutrition and training programs for athletes.

DR MICHAEL COLGAN/SPEAKER

Dr Colgan speaks worldwide to sports, medical and corporate organizations, and is frequently invited to speak at a variety of annual conventions. His fast-moving, informative and entertaining lectures on nutrition, aging and athletic performance, draw capacity audiences in the US, Canada, Britain, Australia and New Zealand.

Dr Colgan is a regular speaker at the Arnold Schwarznegger Classic, the Natural Products Expo, the National Nutritional Foods Association Conventions, USANA Conventions, Tegel Foods, Les Mills Gyms, Nu-Life and the International Association of Clinical Nutritionists.

For further information, or to book Dr Colgan to speak at an event, phone 1-760-632-7722, or visit the Colgan Institute website at www.colgan-institute.com.

References

Chapter One: New Facts, New Focus

1. Centers for Disease Control and Prevention. Impact of arthritis and other rheumatic conditions on the health-care system. **JAMA,** 1999;281:2177.
2. Robbins SI, et al. **Pathologic Basis of Disease,** Philadelphia PA: WB Saunders, 1984:1356-1361.
3. Krupp MA, Chatton MJ, (eds). **Current Medical Treatment and Diagnosis.** Los Altos CA: Large Medical Publications, 1982:487-491.
4. Schumacher, HR. Crystal-induced arthritis: an overview. **AM J Med,** 1996;100:46S-52S.
5. Fam, AG, et al. Gouty arthritis in nodal osteoarthritis. **J Rheumatol,** 1996;23:684-689.
6. Newman NM, Ling RSM. Acetabular bone destruction related to non-steroidal anti-inflammatory drugs. **Lancet,** 1985;2:11-14.
7. Solomon L. Drug-induced arthropathy of the femoral head. **J Bone Joint Surg Br,** 1973;55:246-261.
8. Colgan M. **The New Nutrition: Medicine For The Millennium.** Vancouver: Apple Publishing, 1995.

Chapter Two: Lean and Clean

1. Boyd Eaton S, et al. **The Paleolithic Prescription.** New York: Harper and Row, 1988.
2. Masaro M, et al. Primitive diets of our ancestors. **New Engl J Med,** 1985;31 January:4-8.
3. Lucas P, Power L, Dietary fat aggravates active rheumatoid arthritis. **Clin Res,** 1981;29:754A.
4. Colgan M. **Essential Fats.** Vancouver: Apple Publishing, 1998.
5. Colgan M. **Essential Fats for Athletes**. Vancouver: Apple Publishing, 1998.
6. Ziff M. Diet in the treatment of rheumatoid arthritis. **Arth Rheum,** 1983;26:457-461.

7. Shapiro JA, et al. Diet and rheumatoid arthritis in women: a possible protective effect of fish consumption. **Epidemiol,** 1996;7:256-263.
8. Colgan M. **The New Nutrition: Medicine For The Millennium.** Vancouver: Apple Publishing, 1995.
9. La Vecchia C, et al. Vegetable consumption and risk of chronic disease. **Epidemiol,** 1998;9:208-210.
10. Kjeldsen-Kragh J, et al. Changes in laboratory variables in rheumatoid arthritis patients during a trial of fasting and one-year vegetarian diet. **Scand J Rheumatol,** 1995;24:85-93.
11. Nenonen MT, et al. Uncooked, lactobacilli-rich vegan food and rheumatoid arthritis. **Brit J Rheumatol,** 1998;37:274-281.
12. Colgan M. **Prevent Cancer Now.** San Diego: C.I. Publications, 1992.
13. Klemp P, et al. Gout is on the increase in New Zealand. **Ann Rheum Dis,** 1997;56:22-26.
14. Rubinstein E, Federman DD. **Scientific American Medicine,** New York: Scientific American, 1986;15:1-11.
15. Fam AG, et al. Gouty arthritis in nodal osteoarthritis. **J Rheumatol,** 1996;23:684-689.
16. Schumacher HR. Crystal-induced arthritis: an overview. **Am J Med,** 1996;100:465-525.
17. Yamanaka H. Alcohol ingestion and hyperuricaemia. **Nippon Rinsho,** 1996;54:3369-3373.
18. Faller J, Fox IH. Ethanol-induced hyperuricaemia: evidence for increased urate production by activation of adenine nucleotide turnover. **New Engl J Med,** 1982;307:1598-1602.
19. Eastmond C J, et al. The effects of alcoholic beverages on urate metabolism in gout sufferers. **Br J Rheumatol,** 1995;34:756-759.
20. Emmerson BT. Effect of oral fructose on urate production. **Ann Rheum Dis,** 1974;33:276-280.
21. Colgan M. **Hormonal Health.** Vancouver:Apple Publishing, 1996.
22. Lewis AS, et al. Inhibition of mammalian xanthine oxidase by folate compounds and amethopterin. **J Biol Chem,** 1984;259:12-15.

Chapter Three: Omega-3 Fats Whack Arthritis

1. Colgan M. **Essential Fats.** Vancouver: Apple Publishing, 1998.
2. Budwig J. **Flax Oil as a True Aid Against Arthritis, Heart Infarction, Cancer and Other Diseases.** Vancouver: Apple Publishing, 1992.

3.   Kremer JM, et al. Dietary fish oil and olive oil supplementation in patients with rheumatoid arthritis. Clinical and immunological effects. **Arthritis Rheum,** 1990;33:810-820.
4.   Lau CS, et al. Effects of fish oil supplementation on nonsteroidal anti-inflammatory drug requirement in patients with mild rheumatoid arthritis -- a double-blind, placebo controlled study. **Brit J Rheumatol,** 1993;32:982-989.
5.   Nielsen GL, et al. The effects of dietary supplementation with n–3 polyunsaturated fatty acids in patients with rheumatoid arthritis: randomized double-blind trial. **Eur J Clin Invest,** 1992;22:687-691.
6.   Kremer JM, et al. Effects of high-dose fish oil on rheumatoid arthritis after stopping non-steroidal anti-inflammatory drugs. Clinical and immune correlates. **Arthritis Rheum,** 1995;38:1107-1114.
7.   Cleland LG, James MJ. Rheumatoid arthritis and the balance of dietary N-6 and N-3 essential fatty acids. **Brit J Rheumatol,** 1997;36:513-514.
8.   Shukla VK, Perkins EG. The presence of oxidative polymeric materials in encapsulated fish oils. **Lipids,** 1991;26:23-26.
9.   Mantzioris E, et al. Dietary substitution with an alpha-linolenic acid rich vegetable oil increases eicosapentaenoic acid concentration in tissues. **Am J Clin Nutr,** 1994;59:1304-1309.
10. Kelley DS. Alpha-linolenic acid and immune response. **Nutrition,** 1992;8:215-217.

Chapter Four: Omega-6 Fats Whack Arthritis

1.   Rothman D, et al. Botanical lipids: effects on inflammation, immune responses and rheumatoid arthritis. **Semin Arthritis Rheum,** 1995;25:87-96.
2.   Leventhal LJ, et al. Treatment of rheumatoid arthritis with blackcurrant seed oil. **Brit J Rheumatol,** 1994;33:847-852.
3.   Zurier RB, et al. Gamma-Linoleic acid treatment of rheumatoid arthritis. A randomized, placebo-controlled trial. **Arthritis Rheum,** 1996;39:1808-1817.
4.   Watson J, et al. Cytokine and prostaglandin production by monocytes of volunteers and rheumatoid arthritis patients treated with dietary supplements of blackcurrant seed oil. **Brit J Rheumatol,** 1993;32:1055-1058.

Chapter Five: Essential Fats Combat Inflammation

1. Watson J, et al. Cytokine and prostaglandin production by monocytes of volunteers and rheumatoid arthritis patients treated with dietary supplements of blackcurrant seed oil. **Brit J Rheumatol**, 1993;32:1055-1058.
2. Hughes DA, Pinder AC. Influence of n-3 polyunsaturated fatty acids (PUFA) on the antigen-presenting function of human monocytes. **Biochem Soc Trans**, 1996;24:389s.
3. Kremer JM. Effects of modulation of inflammatory and immune parameters in patients with rheumatic and inflammatory disease receiving dietary supplementation of n-3 and n-6 fatty acids. **Lipids**, 1996;31:Suppl:S243-S247.
4. Rossetti RG, et al. Differential regulation of human T lymphocyte protein kinase C activity by unsaturated fatty acids. **Clin Immunol Immunopathol**, 1995;76:220-224.

Chapter Six: Glucosamine Forms Half The Structure

1. Colgan M. **Optimum Sports Nutrition**. New York: Advanced Research Press, 1993.
2. Setnikar J. Absorption, distribution and excretion of radioactivity after a single intravenous or oral administration of [14C] glucosamine to the rat. **Pharmatherapeutica**, 1984;3:538-550.
3. Setnikar I. Pharmacokinetics of glucosamine in the dog and in man. **Arneimittelforschung**, 1986;36:729-736.
4. Lopez Vaz A. Double-blind clinical evaluation of the relative efficacy of ibuprofen and glucosamine sulfate in the management of osteoarthrosis of the knee in out patients. **Curr Med Res Opin**, 1982;8:145-149.
5. D'Ambrosio E, et al. Glucosamine sulfate: Controlled clinical investigation in arthrosis. **Pharmatherapeutica**, 1981;2:504-508. Bohmen D, et al (eds). Treatment of chondropathia patellae in young athletes with glucosamine sulfate. **Current Topics In Sports Medicine**. Vienna: Urban and Schwarzenberg, 1984.

Chapter Seven: The Chondroitin Dilemma

1. Andermann G, Dietz M. The influence of the route of administration on the bioavailability of an endogenous macromolecule, chondroitin sulfate (CSA). **Eur J Drug Metab Pharm Pharmacokinet,** 1982;7:11-16.
2. Pescador R, Madonna M. Pharmokinetics of fluorescin-labelled glycosaminoglycans and of their lipoprotein lipase-inducing activity in the rat. **Arzneim-Forsch Drug Res,** 1982;32:819-824.
3. Clevidence, BA, et al. Pharmacokinetics of Catalytically Tritiated Glycosaminoglycans in the Rat. **Arzneim-Forsh,** 1983;33(2):228-230.
4. Baici A, et al. Analysis of glycosaminoglycans in human serum after oral administration of chondroitin sulfate. **Rheumatol Int,** 1992;12:81-88.
5. Morreale P, et al. Comparison of the anti-inflammatory efficacy of chondroitin sulfate and diclofenac sodium in patients with knee osteoarthritis. **J Rheumatol,** 1996;23:1385-1391.
6. Conte A, et al. Biochemical and pharmaconkinetic aspects of oral treatment with chondroitin sulfate. **Arzneimittelforschung,** 1995 Aug;45(8):918-925.
7. Silvestro L, et al. Human pharmacokinetics of glycosaminoglycans using deutrium-labeled and unlabeled substances: evidence for oral absorption. **Semin Thromb Hemost** 1994:20:281-292.
8. Gustafson S. The influence of sulfated polysaccharides on the circulating levels of hyaluronan. **Glycobiology,** 1997;7(8):1209-1214.
9. Hutadilok N, et al. **Ther Res,** 1988;44:845.
10. Bassleer C, et al. **Int J Tassne React,** 1992;14:231.
11. McKown KM et al. Lack of efficacy of bovine type II collagen added to existing therapy in rheumatoid arthritis. **Arthritis Rheum,** 1999;42:1204-1208.
12. Leeb BF, et al. Results of multi center study of chondroitin sulfate use in arthroses of the finger, knee and hip joints. **Wien Med Wochenschr,** 1996;146:609-614.

Chapter Eight: SAMe Breakthrough

1. Barcelo HA, et al. Effect of S-adenosylmethionine on experimental osteoarthritis in rabbits. **Am J Med,** 1987;83:55-59.

2. Stramentinoli G. Pharmacological aspects of S-adenosylmethionine. Pharmacokinetics and pharmacodynamics. **Am J Med**, 1987;83:35-42.
3. di Padova C. S-adenosylmethionine in the treatment of osteoarthritis. Review of the clinical studies. **Am J Med**, 1987;83:60-65.
4. Gutierrez S, et al. SAMe restores the changes in the proliferation and in the synthesis of fibronectin and proteoglycans induced by tumour necrosis factor alpha on cultured rabbit synovial cells. **Brit J Rheumatol**, 1997;36:27-31.
5. Muller-Fassbender H. Double-blind clinical trial of S-adenosylmethionine versus ibuprofen in the treatment of osteoarthritis. **Am J Med**, 1987;83:81-83.
6. Caruso I, Pietrogrande V. Italian double-blind multi center study comparing S-adenosylmethionine, naproxen and placebo in the treatment of degenerative joint disease. **Am J Med**, 1987;83:66-71.
7. Vetter G. Double-blind comparative clinical trial with S-adenosylmethionine and indomethacin in the treatment of osteoarthritis. **Am J Med**, 1987;83:78-80.
8. Maccagno A, et al. Double-blind controlled clinical trial of oral S-adenosylmethionine versus piroxicam in knee osteoarthritis. **Am J Med**, 1987;83:72-77.
9. Konig B. A long-term (two years) clinical trial with S-adenosylmethionine for the treatment of osteoarthritis. **Am J Med**, 1987;83:89-94.
10. Tavoni A, et al. Evaluation of S-adenosylmethionine in primary fibromyalgia. A double-blind crossover study. **Am J Med**, 1987;83:107-110.
11. Jacobsen S, et al. Oral S-adenosylmethionine in primary fibromyalgia. Double-blind clinical evaluation. **Scand J Rheumatol**, 1991;20:294-302.

Chapter Nine: The Homocysteine Connection

1. McCully KS. Homocysteine, Folate, Vitamin B_6 and cardiovascular disease. **JAMA**, 1998;279:392-393.
2. Rimm EB, et al. Folate and vitamin B_6 from diet and supplements in relation to risk of coronary heart disease among women. **JAMA**, 1998;279:359-364.

3. Regland B, et al. Increased concentrations of homocysteine in the cerebrospinal fluid in patients with fibromyalgia and chronic fatigue syndrome. **Scand J Rheumatol,** 1997;26:301-307.

4. Parnetti L, et al. Role of homocysteine in age-related vascular and non-vascular diseases. **Aging (Milano),** 1997;9:241-257.

5. Fava M, et al. Folate, vitamin B12 and homocysteine in major depressive disorder. **Am J Psychiat,** 1997;154:426-428.

6. Roubenoff R, et al. Abnormal homocysteine metabolism in rheumatoid arthritis. **Arth Rheum,** 1997;40:718-722.

7. Joosten E, et al. Is metabolic evidence for vitamin B_{12} and folate deficiency more frequent in elderly patients with Alzheimer's disease? **J Gerontol A Biol Sci Med Sci,** 1997;52:M76-79.

8. Bottiglieri T, et al. Folate, vitamin B12 and neuropozehiatine disorders. **Nutr Rev,** 1996;54:382-390.

9. Graham IM, et al. Plasma homocysteine as a risk factor for vascular disease. The European Concerted Action Project. **JAMA,** 1997;277:1775-1781.

10. Ward M, et al. Plasma homocysteine, a risk factor for cardiovascular disease, is lowered by physiological doses of folic acid. **Quar J Med,** 1997;90:519-524.

11. de Bree A, et al. Folate intake in Europe: recommended, actual and desired intake. **Eur J Clin Nutr,** 1997;51:643-660.

12. **US RDA Handbook, 10th Edition.** Washington, DC: National Academy Press, 1989.

13. Bates CJ, et al. Plasma total homocysteine in a representative sample of 972 British men and women aged 65 and over. **Eur J Clin Nutr,** 1997;51:691-697.

14. Stabler SP, et al. Vitamin B-12 deficiency in the elderly: current dilemmas. **Am J Clin Nutr,** 1997;66:741-749.

15. Evers S, et al. Features, symptoms and neurophysiological findings in stroke associated with hyperhomocysteinemia. **Arch Neurol,** 1997;54:1276-1282.

16. Morrison LD, et al. Brain S-adenosylmethionine levels are severely decreased in Alzheimer's disease. **J Neurochem,** 1996;67:1328-1331.

17. Shiroky JB. The use of folates concomitantly with low-dose pulse methotrexate. **Rheum Dis Clin North Am,** 1997;23:969-980.

Chapter Ten: Beating Arthritic Depression

1. Roubenoff R, et al. Abnormal homocysteine metabolism in rheumatoid arthritis. **Arth Rheum**, 1997;40:718-722.
2. Regland B, et al. Increased concentrations of homocysteine in the cerebrospinal fluid in patients with fibromyalgia and chronic fatigue syndrome. **Scand J Rheumatol**, 1997;26:301-307.
3. Parnetti L, et al. Role of homocysteine in age-related vascular and non-vascular diseases. **Aging (Milano)**, 1997;9:241-257.
4. Fava M, et al. Folate, vitamin B12 and homocysteine in major depressive disorder. **Am J Psychiat**, 1997;154:426-428.
5. Joosten E, et al. Is metabolic evidence for vitamin B_{12} and folate deficiency more frequent in elderly patients with Alzheimer's. **J Gerontol A Biol Sci Med Sci**, 1997;52:M76-79.
6. Bottiglieri T, et al. Folate, vitamin B12 and neuropsychiatric disorders. **Nutr Rev**, 1996;54:382-390.
7. Graham IM, et al. Plasma homocysteine as a risk factor for vascular disease. The European Concerted Action Project. **JAMA,** 1997;277:1775-1781.
8. Ward M, et al. Plasma homocysteine, a risk factor for cardiovascular disease, is lowered by physiological doses of folic acid. **Quar J Med,** 1997;90:519-524.
9. Malinow M, et al. Reduction of plasma homocysteine levels by breakfast cereal fortified with folic acid in patients with coronary heart disease. **New Engl J Med,** 1998;338:1009-1015.
10. Moghadasian MH, et al. Homocysteine and coronary artery disease. Clinical evidence and genetic and metabolic background. **Arch Int Med,** 1997;157:2299-2308.
11. Stabler SP, et al. Vitamin B-12 deficiency in the elderly: current dilemmas. **Am J Clin Nutr**, 1997;66:741-749.
12. Loehrer FM, et al. Influence of oral S-adenosylmethionine on plasma 5-methyltetrahydrofolate, S-adenosylhomocysteine, homocysteine and methionine in healthy humans. **J Pharmacol Exp Ther,** 1997;282:845-850.
13. Baldessarini, RJ. Neuropharmacology of S-adenosyl-L-methionine. **Am J Med,** 1987;83:95-103.
14. Morrison LD, et al. Brain S-adenosylmethionine levels are severely decreased in Alzheimer's diseases. **J Neurochem,** 1996;67:1328-1331.

15. Konig B. A long-term (two years) clinical trial with S-adenosylmethionine for the treatment of osteoarthritis. **Am J Med,** 1987;83:89-94.
16. Tavoni A, et al. Evaluation of S-adenosylmethionine in primary fibromyalgia: a double-blind crossover study. **Am J Med,** 1987;83:107-110.
17. Jacobsen S, et al. Oral S-adenosylmethionine in primary fibromyalgia. Double-blind clinical evaluation. **Scand J Rheumatol,** 1991;20:294-302.

Chapter 11: Antioxidants Against Arthritis

1. Harmon D. A theory based on free radical and radiation chemistry. **J Gerontol,** 1956;11:298-300.
2. Kitani K, et al (eds). **Pharmacological Intervention in Aging and Age-Associated Disorders.** New York: New York Academy of Sciences, 1996.
3. Colgan M. **The New Nutrition: Medicine For The Millennium.** Vancouver: Apple Publishing, 1995.
4. Colgan M. **Antioxidants: The Real Story.** Vancouver: Apple Publishing, 1998.
5. Cooper K. **The Antioxidant Revolution.** Nashville: Thomas Nelson, 1994.
6. **USA Today,** 4 March 1994;1A.
7. Chandra, R. Graying of the immune system. Can nutrient supplements improve immunity in the elderly? **JAMA,** 1997;277:1398-1399.
8. Kremer JM, Bigaouette J. Nutrient intake of patients with rheumatoid arthritis is deficient in pyridoxine, zinc, copper, and magnesium. **J Rheumatol,** 1996;23:990-994.
9. Stone J, et al. Inadequate calcium, vitamin E, zinc and selenium intake in rheumatoid arthritis patients: results of a dietary survey. **Semin Arth Rheum,** 1997;27:180-185.
10. Heinle K, et al. Selenium concentration in erythrocytes of patients with rheumatoid arthritis. Clinical and laboratory chemistry infection markers during administration of selenium. **Med Klin,** 1997;92;Suppl 3:29-31.
11. Sklodowska M, et al. Vitamin E, thiobarbituric acid reactive substance concentrations and superoxide dismutase activity in the blood of children with juvenile rheumatoid arthritis. **Clin Exp Rheumatol,** 1996;14:433-439.

12. Morris CJ, et al. Reactive oxygen species and iron –– a dangerous partnership in inflammation. **Int J Biochem Cell Biol**, 1995;27:109-122.
13. Chiriac R, et al. The antioxidant systems in rheumatoid polyarthritis. **Rev Med Chir Soc Med Nat Iasi,** 1996;100:79-83.
14. Comstock GW, et al. Serum concentrations of alpha tocopherol, beta carotene, and retinol preceding the diagnosis of rheumatoid arthritis and systemic lupus erythematosus. **Ann Rheum Dis,** 1997;56:323-325.
15. McAlindon TE, et al. Do antioxidant micronutrients protect against the development and progression of knee osteoarthritis? **Arth Rheum,** 1996;39:648-656.
16. De la Cruz JP, et al. Effects of S-adenosyl-L-methionine on blood platelet activation. **Gen Pharmacol**, 1997;29:651-655.
17. Evans PJ, et al. Antioxidant properties of S-adenosyl-l-methionine: a proposed addition to organ storage fluids. **Free Radic Biol Med**, 1997;23:1002-1008.

Chapter 12: The Hormone Solution

1. Colgan M. **Hormonal Health**. Vancouver: Apple Publishing, 1996.
2. Lahita RG. The connective tissue diseases and the overall influence of gender. **Int J Fertil Menopausal Stud**, 1996;41:156-165.
3. Wilder RL. Adrenal and gonadal steroid hormone deficiency in the pathogenesis of rheumatoid arthritis. **J Rheumatol Suppl**, 1996;44:10-12.
4. Flaisler F, et al. A study of ovarian function in rheumatoid arthritis. **Rev Rheum Engl Ed**, 1995;62:549-554.
5. Lindsay R, Cosman F. Estrogen in prevention and treatment of osteoporosis. **Ann NY Acad Sci**, 1990;592:326-333.
6. Cortet B, et al. Bone tissue in rheumatoid arthritis (2). Pathophysiologic data, pathologic findings, and therapeutic implications. **Rev Rhum Engl Ed**, 1995;62:205-211.
7. Oliveria SA, et al. Estrogen replacement therapy and the development of osteoarthritis. **Epidemiology**, 1996;7:415-419.
8. Spector TD. Is hormone replacement therapy protective for hand and knee osteoarthritis in women?: The Chingford Study. **Ann Rheum Dis**, 1997;56:432-434.
9. Nevitt MC, et al. Association of estrogen replacement therapy with the risk of osteoarthritis of the hip in elderly white women. Study of Osteoporotic Fractures Research Group. **Arch Intern Med**, 1996;156:2073-2080.

10. Siegmeth W, et al. Hormonal status of the woman and its effect on symptoms and progression of chronic polyarthritis. **Acta Med Austriaca,** 1996;23:124-128.

11. Detre T, et al. Management of the Menopause. **Ann Intern Med,** 1978;88:373-378.

12. Calafi Alsina J. Benefits of hormone replacment therapy - overview and update. **Int J Fertil Womens Med,** 1997;42:Suppl 2:329-346.

13. Nachtigall L. **Estrogen: The Facts Can Change Your Life.** New York: Harper/Collins, 1994.

14. Maoz B, Durst N. The effects of estrogen therapy on the sex life of post-menopausal women. **Maturitas,** 1980;2:327-336.

15. Holland EF, et al. Changes in collagen composition and cross-links in bone and skin of osteoporotic postmenopausal women treated with percutaneous estradiol implants. **Obstet Gynecol,** 1994;83:180-183.

16. Maheux R, et al. A randomized, double-blind, placebo-controlled study on the effect of conjugated estrogens on skin thickness. **Am J Obstet Gynecol,** 1994;170:642-649.

17. Havsteen B. Flavonoids, a class of natural products of high pharmacological potency. **Biochem Pharm Pharmacol,** 1983;32:1141-1148.

18. Longcope C, et al. Steroid and gonadotropin levels in women during the peri-menopausal years, **Maturitas,** 1986;8:189-196.

19. Rannevik G, et al. A prospective long-term study in women from pre-menopause to post-menopause: changing profiles of gonadotropins, oestrogens and androgens. **Maturitas,** 1986;8:297-307.

20. Sherwin BB. Affective changes with estrogen and androgen replacement therapy in surgically menopausal women. **J Affect Disord,** 1988;14:177-187.

21. Mirone L, et al. A study of serum androgen and cortisol levels in female patients with rheumatoid arthritis. Correlation with disease activity. **Clin Rheumatol,** 1996;15:15-19

22. Liang MH, Karlson EW. Female hormone therapy and the risk of developing or exacerbating systemic lupus erythematosus or rheumatoid arthritis. **Proc Assoc Am Physicians,** 1996;108:25-28.

23. Nielsen FH, et al. Effect of dietary boron on mineral, estrogen and testosterone metabolism. **FASEB J,** 1987;1:394-397.

24. Sanchez-Capelo A, et al. Potassium regulates plasma testosterone and renal ornithine decarboxylase in mice. **FEBS Lett,** 1993;333:32-34.

25. Hunt CD, et al. Effects of dietary zinc depletion on seminal volume and zinc loss, serum testosterone concentrations and sperm morphology in young men. **Am J Clin Nutr,** 1992;56:148-157.

26. Holden RJ. The estrogen connection: the etilogical relationship between diabetes, cancer, rheumatoid arthritis and psychiatric disorders. **Med Hypotheses**, 1995;45:169-189.
27. Duker EM, et al. Effects of extracts from Cimicifuga racemosa on gonadotropin release in menopausal women and ovariectomized rats. **Planta Med**, 1991;57:420-424.
28. Leonbart JH, et al. **Clin Endocrinol**, 1994;102:448-454.
29. Knight DC, Eden JA. Phytoestrogens - a short review. **Maturitas**, 1995;22:167-175.
30. Washburn SA. A dietary supplement as post-menopausal hormone replacement therapy. **Third International Conference on Phytoestrogens**, Little Rock, AR, December, 1995.
31. Messina MJ, et al. Soy intake and cancer risk: a review of the in vitro and in vivo data. **Nutr Cancer**, 1994;21:113-131.
32. Anderson JW, et al. Meta-analysis of the effects of soy protein intake on serum lipids. **New Engl J Med**, 1995;333:276-282.

Chapter 13: The Road To Happy Joints

1. Colgan M. **The New Nutrition: Medicine For The Millennium.** Vancouver: Apple Publishing, 1995
2. Decker E. Antioxidant activity of whey. Paper presented to the 1997 International Whey Conference, Chicago, Illinois, 1997.
3. Colgan M. **The Sports Nutrition Pocket Guide.** Vancouver: Apple Publishing, 1999.
4. Colgan M. **Optimum Sports Nutrition**. New York: Advanced Research Press, 1993.

Chapter 14: Use It Or Lose It

1. Rall LC, et al. The effect of progressive resistance training in rheumatoid arthritis. Increased strength without changes in energy balance or body composition. **Arthritis Rheum**, 1996;39:415-426.
2. Schilke JM, et al. Effects of muscle-strength training on the functional status of patients with osteoarthritis of the knee joint. **Nurs Res,** 1996;45:68-72.

3. Komatireddy GR, et al. Efficacy of low load resistive muscle training in patients with rheumatoid arthritis functional class II and III. **J Rheumatol**, 1997;24:1531-1539.

4. van den Ende CH, et al. Comparison of high and low intensity training in well controlled rheumatoid arthritis. Results of a randomised clinical trial. **Ann Rheum Dis**, 1996;55:798-805.

5. Ettinger WH Jr, et al. A randomized trial comparing aerobic exercise and resistance exercise with a health education program in older adults with knee osteoarthritis. The Fitness Arthritis and Seniors Trial (FAST). **JAMA**, 1997;277:25-31.

6. Viitanen JV, et al. Fifteen months' follow-up of intensive inpatient physiotherapy and exercise in ankylosing spondylitis. **Clin Rheumatol**, 1995;14:413-419.

7. Neuberger GB, et al. Effects of exercise on fatigue, aerobic fitness, and disease activity measures in persons with rheumatoid arthritis. **Res Nurs Health**, 1997;20:195-204.

8. Prevalence of leisure-time physical activity among persons with arthritis and other rheumatic conditions--United States,1990-1991. **MMWR Morb Mortal Wkly Rep**, 1997;46:389-93.

9. O'Reilly S, et al. Muscle weakness in osteoarthritis. **Curr Opin Rheumatol**, 1997;9:259-262.

10. Tan J, et al. Isokinetic and isometric strength in osteoarthritis of the knee. A comparative study with healthy women. **Am J Phys Med Rehabil**, 1995;74:364-369.

11. Fiatarone MA, et al. Exercise training and nutritional supplementation for physical frailty in very elderly people. **New Engl J Med**, 1994;330:1769-1775.

12. Colgan M. **The New Nutrition: Medicine For The Millennium.** Vancouver: Apple Publications, 1995.

13. Colgan M. **Optimum Sports Nutrition.** New York: Advanced Research Press, 1993.

14. Colgan M. **The Power Program**. Vancouver: Apple Publishing, 1999.

Index

Q

R

S